Third Edition

DRUG CALCULATIONS FOR NURSES

A STEP-BY-STEP APPROACH

Third Edition

DRUG CALCULATIONS FOR NURSES

A STEP-BY-STEP APPROACH

ROBERT LAPHAM BPharm Clin Dip Pharm MRPharmS
Clinical Pharmacist, Sunderland Royal Hospital, City
Hospitals Sunderland NHS Trust, UK

HEATHER AGAR RGN BSc (HONS)
Rheumatology Specialist Nurse, Northumbria Healthcare
NHS Trust, UK

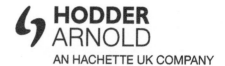
HODDER
ARNOLD
AN HACHETTE UK COMPANY

CRC Press
Taylor & Francis Group, LLC
6000 Broken Sound Parkway NW, Suite 300
Boca Raton, FL 33487-2742

© 2009 by Robert Lapham and Heather Agar
CRC Press is an imprint of Taylor & Francis Group, an Informa business

No claim to original U.S. Government works
Printed on acid-free paper by CPI Group (UK) Ltd, Croydon, CR0 4YY
International Standard Book Number: 978-0-340-98733-9 (Softcover)

**Library of Congress Cataloging-in-Publication Data and
The British Library Cataloging in Publication Data are Available**

**Visit the Taylor & Francis Web site at
http://www.taylorandfrancis.com**

**and the CRC Press Web site at
http://www.crcpress.com**

Poison is in everything, and no thing is without poison. The dosage makes it either a poison or a remedy.

Paracelsus (1493–1541)

Medieval physician and alchemist

Contents

Preface

Drug treatments given to patients in hospital are becoming increasingly complex. Sometimes, these treatment regimes involve potent and, at times, new and novel drugs. Many of these drugs are toxic or possibly fatal if administered incorrectly or in overdose. It is therefore very important to be able to carry out drug calculations correctly so as not to put the patient at risk.

In current nursing practice, the need to calculate drug dosages is not uncommon. These calculations have to be performed competently and accurately, so as not to put not only the nurse but, more importantly, the patient at risk. This book aims to provide an aid to the basics of mathematics and drug calculations. It is intended to be of use to nurses of all grades and specialities, and to be a handy reference for use on the ward.

The concept of this book arose from nurses themselves; a frequently asked question was: 'Can you help me with drug calculations?' Consequently, a small booklet was written to help nurses with their drug calculations, particularly those studying for their IV certificate. This was very well received, and copies were being produced from original copies, indicating the need for such help and a book like this.

The content of the book was determined by means of a questionnaire, sent to nurses asking them what they would like to see featured in a drug calculations book. As a result, this book was written and, hopefully, covers the topics that nurses would like to see.

Although this book was primarily written with nurses in mind, others who use drug calculations in their work will also find it useful. Some topics have been dealt with in greater detail for this reason, e.g. moles and millimoles. This book can be used by anyone who wishes to improve their skills in drug calculations or to use it as a refresher course.

This book is designed to be used for self-study. Before you start, you should attempt the pre-test to assess your current ability in carrying out drug calculations. After completing the book, repeat the same test and compare the two scores to measure your improvement.

To attain maximum benefit from the book, start at the beginning and work through one chapter at a time, as subsequent chapters increase in difficulty. For each chapter attempted, you should understand it a fully and be able to answer the problems confidently before moving on to the next chapter.

Alternatively, if you wish to quickly skip through any chapter, you can refer to the 'Key Points' found at the start of each chapter.

A note about drug names

In the past, the British Approved Name (BAN) was used for drugs in the UK. European law now requires use of the Recommended International Non-proprietary Name (rINN) for medicinal substances. In most cases, the old BAN and the new rINN are identical. Where the two differ, the BAN has been modified to the new rINN; for example: amoxicillin instead of amoxycillin.

Adrenaline and noradrenaline have two names (BAN and rINN). However, adrenaline and noradrenaline are the terms used in the titles of monographs in the *European Pharmacopoeia* and are thus the official names in the member states. The *British Pharmacopoeia 2008* shows the *European Pharmacopoeia* names first followed by the rINN at the head of its monographs (adrenaline/epinephrine); the *British National Formulary* (BNF) has adopted a similar style.

For a full list of all the name changes, see the current edition of the BNF. Affected drugs that appear in this book will be referred to by their new name (rINN) followed by their old name (BAN) in brackets; for adrenaline, this book will follow the convention used by the *British Pharmacopoeia*.

Case reports

The journal *Pharmacy in Practice* highlights real-life medication errors to act as learning points for practitioners. Some of these have been used as Case Reports in this book to illustrate important points to remember.

To obtain the maximum benefit from this book, it is a good idea to attempt the pre-test before you start working through the chapters. The aim of this pre-test is to assess your ability at various calculations.

The pre-test is divided into several sections that correspond to each chapter in the book, and the questions try to reflect the topics covered by each chapter. You don't have to attempt questions for every chapter, only the ones that you feel are relevant to you. Answering the questions will help you identify particular calculations you have difficulty with.

You can use calculators or anything else you find helpful to answer the questions, but it is best to complete the pre-test on your own, as it is **your** ability that is being assessed and not someone else's.

Don't worry if you can't answer all of the questions. As stated before, the aim is to help you to identify areas of weakness. Once again, you don't have to complete every section of the pre-test, just the ones you want to test your ability on.

Once you have completed the pre-test and checked your answers, you can then start working through the chapters. Concentrate particularly on the areas you were weak on and miss out the chapters you were confident with if you wish.

It is up to you as how you use this book, but hopefully the pre-test will help you to identify areas you need to concentrate on.

The pre-test consists of 50 questions and covers all the topics and types of questions in the book. Mark your score out of 50, then double it to find your percentage result.

BASICS

The aim of this section is to test your ability on basic principles such as multiplication, division, fractions, decimals, powers and using calculators, before you start any drug calculations.

Long multiplication

Solve the following:

1 678×465
2 308×1.28

Long division

Solve the following:

3 $3143 \div 28$
4 $37.5 \div 1.25$

Fractions

Solve the following, leaving your answer as a fraction:

5 $\dfrac{5}{9} \times \dfrac{3}{7}$

6 $\dfrac{3}{4} \times \dfrac{12}{16}$

7 $\dfrac{3}{4} \div \dfrac{9}{16}$

8 $\dfrac{5}{6} \div \dfrac{3}{8}$

Convert to a decimal (give answers to 2 decimal places):

9 $\dfrac{2}{5}$

10 $\dfrac{9}{16}$

Decimals

Solve the following:

11 25×0.45
12 $5 \div 0.2$
13 1.38×100
14 $25.64 \div 1{,}000$

Convert the following to a fraction:

15 1.2
16 0.375

Roman numerals

Write the following as ordinary numbers:

17 VII
18 IX

Powers

Convert the following to a proper number:

19 3×10^4

Convert the following number to a power of 10:

20 5,000,000

PER CENT AND PERCENTAGES

This section is designed to see if you understand the concept of per cent and percentages.

21 How much is 28% of 250 g?
22 What percentage is 160 g of 400 g?

UNITS AND EQUIVALENCES

This section is designed to test your knowledge of units normally used in clinical medicine, and how to convert from one unit to another. It is important that you can convert between units easily, as this is the basis for most drug calculations.

Convert the following.

Units of weight

23 0.0625 milligrams (mg) to micrograms (mcg)
24 600 grams (g) to kilograms (kg)
25 50 nanograms (ng) to micrograms (mcg)

Units of volume

26 0.15 litres (L) to millilitres (mL)

Units of amount of substance

Usually describes the amount of electrolytes, as in an infusion (see Chapter 7 'Moles and millimoles' for a full explanation).

27 0.36 moles (mol) to millimoles (mmol)

DRUG STRENGTHS OR CONCENTRATIONS

This section is designed to see if you understand the various ways in which drug strengths can be expressed.

Percentage concentration

28 How much sodium (in grams) is there in a 500 mL infusion of sodium chloride 0.9%?

mg/mL concentrations

29 You have a 5 mL ampoule of dopexamine 1%. How many milligrams of dopexamine are there in the ampoule?

'I in ...' concentrations or ratio strengths

30 You have a 10 mL ampoule of adrenaline/epinephrine 1 in 10,000. How much adrenaline/epinephrine – in milligrams – does the ampoule contain?

Parts per million (ppm) strengths

31 If drinking water contains 0.7 ppm of fluoride, how much fluoride (in milligrams) would be present in 1 litre of water?

DOSAGE CALCULATIONS

These are the types of calculation you will be doing every day on the ward. They include dosages based on patient parameters and paediatric calculations.

Calculating the number of tablets or capsules required

The strength of the tablets or capsules you have available does not always correspond to the dose required. Therefore you have to calculate the number of tablets or capsules needed.

32 The dose prescribed is furosemide (frusemide) 120 mg. You have 40 mg tablets available. How many tablets do you need?

Drug dosage

Sometimes the dose is given on a body weight basis or in terms of body surface area. The following questions test your ability at calculating doses based on these parameters.

Work out the dose required for the following:

33 Dose = 0.5 mg/kg   Weight = 64 kg
34 Dose = 3 mcg/kg/min   Weight = 73 kg
35 Dose = 1.5 mg/m^2 Surface area = 1.55 m^2 (give answer to 3 decimal places)

Calculating dosages

Calculate how much you need for the following dosages:

36 You have aminophylline injection 250 mg in 10 mL.
Amount required = 350 mg
37 You have digoxin injection 500 mcg/2 mL.
Amount required = 0.75 mg
38 You have morphine sulphate elixir 10 mg in 5 mL.
Amount required = 15 mg
39 You have gentamicin injection 40 mg/mL, 2 mL ampoules.
Amount required = 4 mg/kg for a 74 kg patient: how many ampoules will you need?

Paediatric calculations

40 You need to give trimethoprim to a 7-year-old child weighing 23 kg at a dose of 4 mg/kg twice a day.
Trimethoprim suspension comes as a 50 mg in 5 mL suspension.
How much do you need for each dose?

Other factors to take into account are displacement volumes for antibiotic injections.

41 You need to give benzylpenicillin at a dose of 200 mg to a 6-month-old baby. The displacement volume for benzylpenicillin is 0.4 mL per 600 mg vial.
How much water for injections do you need to add to ensure a strength of 600 mg per 5 mL?

MOLES AND MILLIMOLES

This section is designed to see if you understand the concept of millimoles. Millimoles are used to describe the 'amount of substance', and are usually the units for body electrolytes (e.g. sodium 138 mmol/L).

Moles and millimoles

42 Approximately how many millimoles of sodium are there in a 10 mL ampoule of sodium chloride 30% injection? (Molecular mass of sodium chloride = 58.5)

Molarity

43 How many grams of sodium chloride is required to make 200 ml of a 0.5 M solution? (Molecular mass of sodium chloride = 58.5)

INFUSION RATE CALCULATIONS

This section tests your knowledge of various infusion rate calculations. It is designed to see if you know the different drop factors for different giving sets and fluids, as well as being able to convert volumes to drops and vice versa.

Calculation of drip rates

44 What is the rate required to give 500 mL of sodium chloride 0.9% infusion over 6 hours using a standard giving set?
45 What is the rate required to give 1 unit of blood (500 mL) over 8 hours using a standard giving set?

Conversion of dosages to mL/hour

Sometimes it may be necessary to convert a dose (mg/min) to an infusion rate (mL/hour).

46 You have an infusion of dopamine 800 mg in 500 mL. The dose required is 2 mcg/kg/min for a patient weighing 60 kg.
   What is the rate in mL/hour?

47 You are asked to give 500 mL of doxapram 0.2% infusion at a rate of 3 mg/min using an infusion pump.
   What is the rate in mL/hour?

Conversion of mL/hour back to a dose

48 You have dopexamine 50 mg in 50 mL and the rate at which the pump is running is 21 mL/hour. What dose – in mcg/kg/min – is the pump delivering?
   (Patient's weight = 88 kg)

Calculating the length of time for IV infusions

49 A 500 mL infusion of sodium chloride 0.9% is being given at a rate of 21 drops/min (standard giving set).
   How long will the infusion run at the specified rate?

50 A 250 mL infusion of sodium chloride 0.9% is being given at a rate of 42 mL/hour.
   How long will the infusion run at the specified rate?

ANSWERS

1 315,270
2 394.24
3 112.25
4 30
5 $\dfrac{5}{21}$
6 $\dfrac{9}{16}$
7 $\dfrac{4}{3}$
8 $\dfrac{20}{9}$
9 0.40
10 0.56 (0.5625)
11 11.25
12 25

13 138

14 0.02564

15 $\frac{6}{5}$

16 $\frac{3}{8}$

17 7

18 9

19 30,000

20 5×10^6

21 70 g

22 40%

23 62.5 micrograms

24 0.6 kilograms

25 0.05 micrograms

26 150 millilitres

27 360 millimoles

28 4.5 g

29 50 milligrams

30 1 mg

31 0.7 mg

32 Three furosemide (frusemide) 40 mg tablets

33 32 mg

34 219 mcg/min

35 2.325 mg

36 14 mL

37 3 mL

38 7.5 mL

39 4 ampoules

40 9.2 mL

41 4.6 mL

42 51.3 mmol (rounded to 51 mmol)

Sometimes it is necessary to adjust the dose by rounding like this for ease of calculation and administration, as long as the adjustment is not so much that it makes a large difference to the amount.

43 5.85 g sodium chloride

44 27.7 drops/min (rounded to 28 drops/min)

45 15.625 drops/min (rounded to 16 drops/min)

46 4.5 mL/hour

47 90 mL/hour

48 3.98 mcg/kg/min (approx. 4 mcg/kg/min)

49 7.94 hours (approx. 8 hours)

50 5.95 hours (approx. 6 hours)

PART 1: Mathematics

1 FIRST PRINCIPLES

OBJECTIVES

At the end of this chapter, you should be familiar with the following:

- Sense of number and working from first principles
- Estimation of answers
- The 'ONE unit' rule
- Checking your answer – does it seem reasonable?
- Minimizing errors

BEFORE WE START

Drug calculation questions are a major concern for most healthcare professionals, including nurses and those teaching them. There have been numerous articles highlighting the poor performance of various healthcare professionals.

The vast majority of calculations are likely to be relatively straightforward and you will probably not need to perform any complex calculation very often. But it is obvious that people are struggling with basic calculations.

It is difficult to explain why people find maths difficult, but the best way to overcome this is to try to make maths easy to understand by going back to first principles. The aim is not to demean or offend anyone, but to recall and explain the basics. Maths is just another language that tells us how we measure and estimate, and these are the two key words.

It is vital, however, that any person performing dose calculations using any method, formula or calculator can understand and explain how the final dose is actually arrived at through the calculation.

SENSE OF NUMBER AND WORKING FROM FIRST PRINCIPLES

There is a risk that calculators and formulae can be used without a basic understanding of what exactly the numbers being entered actually mean; consequently there is a potential for mistakes. Working from first principles and using basic arithmetical skills allows you to have a 'sense of number' and in doing so reduces the risk of making mistakes.

Indeed, the NMC *Standards for Medicines Management* (2008) states:

> The use of calculators to determine the volume or quantity of medication should not act as a substitute for arithmetical knowledge and skill.

To ensure that when pharmacists qualify they have basic arithmetical skills and this 'sense of number', the Royal Pharmaceutical Society of Great Britain has banned the use of calculators from their registration exam. However, this is not to say that calculators should not be used – calculators can increase accuracy and can be helpful for complex calculations.

The main problem with using a calculator or a formula is the belief that it is infallible and that the answer it gives is right and can be taken to be true without a second thought. This infallibility is, to some extent, true, but it certainly does not apply to the user; the adage 'rubbish in equals rubbish out' certainly applies.

An article that appeared in the *Nursing Standard* in May 2008 also highlighted the fact that using formulae relies solely on arithmetic and gives answers that are devoid of meaning and context. The article mentions that skill is required to: extract the correct numbers from the clinical situation; place them correctly in the formula; perform the arithmetic; and translate the answer back to the clinical context to find the meaning of the number and thence the action to be taken.

How can you be certain that the answer you get is correct if you have no 'sense of number'? You have no means of knowing whether the numbers have been entered correctly – you may have entered them the wrong way round.

For example, if when calculating 60 per cent of 2 you enter:

$$\frac{100}{60} \times 2 \text{ instead of } \frac{60}{100} \times 2$$

You would get an answer of 3.3 instead of the correct answer of 1.2. If you have a 'sense of number' you would immediately realize that the answer 3.3 is wrong.

Another advantage of working from first principles is that you can put your answer back into the correct clinical context.

You may have entered the numbers correctly into your formula and calculator and arrived at the correct answer of 1.2 – but what does it mean? You might mistakenly believe that you need to give 1.2 ampoules instead of 1.2 mL. If so, you would need to work out the volume to be drawn up which equals 1.2 ampoules – more calculations and more potential mistakes!

All this may seem unbelievable – but these things do happen.

References

NMC. *Standards for Medicine Management* (2008). Nursing and Midwifery Council, London.

K Wright. Drug calculations part 1: a critique of the formula used by nurses. *Nursing Standard* 2008; **22** (36): 40–42.

ESTIMATION OF ANSWERS

Looking at a drug calculation with a 'sense of number' means that we can often have a 'rough idea' or estimate of the answer.

Simple techniques of halving, doubling, addition and multiplication can be used. For example:

1 You have: 200 mg in 10 mL
  From this, you can easily work out the following equivalents:
  100 mg in 5 mL (by halving)
  50 mg in 2.5 mL (by halving again)
  150 mg in 7.5 mL (by addition: 100 mg + 50 mg and 5 mL + 2.5 mL)
2 You have: 100 mg in 1 mL
  From this, you can easily work out the following:
  500 mg in 5 mL (by addition: 100 mg + 100 mg + 100 mg + 100 mg + 100 mg and 1 mL + 1 mL + 1 mL + 1 mL + 1 mL)
  500 mg in 5 mL (by multiplication: 100 mg × 5 and 1 mL × 5)
  200 mg in 2 mL (by doubling)

If estimation is not possible, then rely on experience and common sense. If your answer means that you would need six ampoules of an injection for your calculated dose, then common sense should dictate that this is not normal practice (see later: 'Checking your answer – does it seem reasonable?').

THE 'ONE UNIT' RULE

Various methods are available for drug calculations – we will be using the 'ONE unit' rule throughout this book. Using it will enable you to work from first principles and have a 'sense of number'.

The rule works by proportion: what you do to one side of an equation, do the same to the other side. In whatever the type of calculation you are doing, it is always best to make what you've got equal to **one** and then multiply by what you want – hence the name.

The following example will explain the concept more clearly. We will use boxes in the form of a table to make the explanation easier.

If 12 apples cost £2.88, how much would 5 apples cost?

If we have a 'sense of number' we can estimate our answer. Six apples would cost half of £2.88 which would be £1.44; 3 apples would cost half of that: 72p. So 5 apples would cost between 72p and £1.44; probably nearer the upper figure – say £1.20, as a guess.

Now let's do the calculation using the 'ONE unit' rule:
Write down everything we know:

   12 apples   cost   £2.88

Then write down what we want to know underneath:

   12 apples   cost   £2.88
    5 apples   cost   ?

We will write everything using boxes in the form of a table:

L		R
12 apples	cost	£2.88
5 apples	cost	?

The left-hand side (column L) = what you know and what you want to know.

The right-hand side (column R) = the known and unknown.

First calculate how much **one** of whatever you have (ONE unit) is equal to. This is done by proportion. Make everything you know (the left-hand side or column L) equal to 1 by dividing by 12:

$$\frac{12}{12}\text{apples} = 1 \text{ apple}$$

As we have done this to one side of the equation (column L), we must do the same to the other side (column R):

$$\frac{£2.88}{12}$$

L		R
12 apples	cost	£2.88
apples = 1 apple	cost	

Next, multiply by what you want to know; in this case it is the cost of 5 apples.

So multiply 1 apple (column L) by 5 and don't forget, we have to do the same to the other side of the equation (right-hand side or column R):

L	R	
12 apples	cost	£2.88
$\dfrac{12}{12}$ apples = 1 apple	cost	$\dfrac{£2.88}{12}$
5 apples = 1 × 5 = 5	cost	$\dfrac{£2.88}{12} × 5 = £1.20$

So 5 apples would cost £1.20.

Working from first principles ensures that the correct units are used and that there is no confusion as to what the answer actually means.

Checking with our original estimation: 5 apples would cost between 72p to £1.44; probably nearer the upper figure – say £1.20, as a guess.

Our guess was the correct answer.

The above is a lengthy way of doing a simple calculation. In reality, we would have completed the calculation in three steps:

$$12 \text{ apples cost } £2.88$$

$$1 \text{ apple cost } \dfrac{£2.88}{12}$$

$$5 \text{ apples cost } \dfrac{£2.88}{12} × 5 = £1.20$$

CHECKING YOUR ANSWER: DOES IT SEEM REASONABLE?

As stated before, it is good practice to have a rough idea of the answer first, so you can check your final calculated answer. Your estimate can be a single value or, more usually, a range in which your answer should fall. If the answer you get is outside this range, then your answer is wrong and you should re-check your calculations.

The following guide may be useful in helping you to decide whether your answer is reasonable or not. Any answer outside these ranges probably means that you have calculated the wrong answer.

The maximum you should give a patient for any one dose:

TABLETS   Not more than 4*
LIQUIDS   Anything from 5 mL to 20 mL
INJECTIONS Anything from 1 mL to 10 mL

*An exception to this would be prednisolone. Some doses of prednisolone may mean the patient taking up to 10 tablets at any one time. Even with prednisolone, it is important to check the dose and the number of tablets.

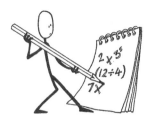

Always write your calculations down

PUTTING IT ALL TOGETHER

Using all the above principles, consider the following situation: you have an injection of pethidine with the strength of 100 mg per 2 mL and you need to give a dose of 60 mg.

First – have a rough idea of your answer by estimation. By looking at what you have – 100 mg in 2 mL – you can assume the following:

- The dose you want (60 mg) will be
  - less than 2 mL (2 mL = 100 mg)
  - more than 1 mL (1 mL = 50 mg – by halving)
  - less than 1.5 mL (0.5 mL = 25 mg – by halving and addition: 1 mL + 0.5 mL = 75 mg)
  - less than 1.25 mL (0.25 mL = 12.5 mg – by halving and addition: 1 + 0.25 mL = 62.5 mg)
- From the above, you would estimate that your answer would be within the range 1–1.25 mL.

Calculate from first principles – using the 'ONE unit' rule:

$$100\,mg = 2\,mL$$

$$1\,mg = \frac{2}{100}\,mL$$

$$60\,mg = \frac{2}{100} \times 60 = 1.2\,mL$$

Working from first principles, you derive an answer of 1.2 mL. This is within your estimated range of 1–1.25 mL.

Does your answer seem reasonable? The answer is yes. It correlates to your estimation and only a part of the ampoule will be used which, from common sense, seems reasonable.

MINIMIZING ERRORS

- Write out the calculation clearly. It is all too easy to end up reading from the wrong line.
  If you are copying formulae from a reference source, double-check what you have written down.
- Write down every step.
- Remember to include the units at every step; this will avoid any confusion over what your answer actually means.
- Do not take short cuts; you are more likely to make a mistake.
- Try not to be totally dependent on your calculator. Have an approximate idea of what the answer should be. Then, if you happen to hit the wrong button on the calculator you are more likely to be aware that an error has been made.
- Finally, always double-check your calculation. There is frequently more than one way of doing a calculation, so if you get the same answer by two different methods the chances are that your answer will be correct. Alternatively, try working it in reverse and see if you get the numbers you started with.

REMEMBER

If you are in any doubt about a calculation you are asked to do on the ward – **stop** and get help.

2 BASICS

OBJECTIVES

At the end of this chapter, you should be familiar with the following:

- Arithmetic symbols
- Basic maths
  Long multiplication
  Long division
  Mathematical tips and tricks
- Rules of arithmetic
- Fractions and decimals
  Reducing or simplifying fractions
  Equivalent fractions
  Adding and subtracting fractions
  Multiplying fractions
  Dividing fractions
  Converting fractions to decimals
  Multiplying decimals
  Dividing decimals
  Rounding of decimal numbers
  Converting decimals to fractions
- Roman numerals
- Powers or exponentials
- Using a calculator
- Powers and calculators
- Estimating answers

KEY POINTS

Basic Arithmetic Rules

- Simple basic rules exist when adding (+), subtracting (−), multiplying (×) and dividing (/ or ÷) numbers − these are known as operations.
- The acronym or word BEDMAS can be used to remember the correct order of operations:

B	Do calculations in **brackets** first. When you have more than one set of brackets, do the inner brackets first.
E	Next, do any **exponentiation** (or powers).
D and **M**	Do the **division** and **multiplication** in order from left to right.
A and **S**	Do the **addition** and **subtraction** in order from left to right.

Fractions

• A fraction consists of a **numerator** and a **denominator**:

$$\frac{\text{numerator}}{\text{denominator}} \quad \text{e.g.} \quad \frac{2}{5}$$

• With calculations, it is best to try to simplify or reduce fractions to their **lowest terms**.
• **Equivalent fractions** are those with the same value, e.g. $\frac{1}{2}, \frac{3}{6}, \frac{4}{8}, \frac{12}{24}$. If you reduce them to their simplest form, you will notice that each is exactly a half.
• If you want to convert fractions to equivalent fractions with the **same** denominator, you have to find a common number that is divisible by all the individual denominators.

Operations with fractions

• To add (or subtract) fractions with the **same** denominator, add (or subtract) the numerators and place the result over the common denominator.
• To add (or subtract) fractions with the **different** denominators, first convert them to equivalent fractions with the same denominator, then add (or subtract) the numerators and place the result over the common denominator as before.
• To multiply fractions, multiply the numerators and the denominators.
• To divide fractions, invert the second fraction and multiply (as above).
• To convert a fraction to a decimal, divide the numerator by the denominator.

Decimals

• When multiplying or dividing decimals, ensure that the decimal point is placed in the correct place.
• Rounding decimals up or down:

    If the number after the decimal point is **4 or less**, then ignore it, i.e. **round down**;

    If the number after the decimal point is **5 or more**, then add 1 to the whole number, i.e. **round up**.

Roman Numerals

• In Roman numerals, letters are used to designate numbers.

Powers or Exponentials

• Powers or exponentials are a convenient way of writing large or small numbers:

    A positive power or exponent (e.g. 10^5) means **multiply** the base number by itself the number times of the power or exponent

    A negative power or exponent (e.g. 10^{-5}) means **divide** the base number by itself the number of times of the power or exponent.

Using a Calculator

• Ensure that numbers are entered correctly when using a calculator; if necessary, read the manual.

Estimating Answers
- Numbers are either rounded up or down to the nearest ten, hundred or thousand to give numbers that can be calculated easily.
- Don't forget – the answer is only an estimate.
- If you round up numbers, the estimated answer will be **more** than the actual answer.
- If you round down numbers, the estimated answer will be **less** than the actual answer.

INTRODUCTION

Before dealing with any drug calculations, we will briefly go over a few basic mathematical concepts that may be helpful in some calculations.

This chapter is designed for those who might want to refresh their memories, particularly those who are returning to healthcare after a long absence.

You can simply skip some parts, or all, of this chapter. Alternatively, you can refer back to any part of this chapter as you are working through the rest of the book.

ARITHMETIC SYMBOLS

The following is a table of mathematical symbols generally used in textbooks. The list is not exhaustive, but covers common symbols you may come across.

SYMBOL	MEANING
+	plus or positive; add in calculations
−	minus or negative; subtract in calculations
±	plus or minus; positive or negative
×	multiply by
/ or ÷	divide by
=	equal to
≠	not equal to
≡	identically equal to
≈	approximately equal to
>	greater than
<	less than
≯	not greater than
≮	not less than
≤	equal to or less than
≥	equal to or greater than
%	per cent
Σ	sum of

BASIC MATHS

As a refresher, we will look at basic maths. This is quite useful if you don't have a calculator handy and to understand how to perform drug calculations from first principles.

First, we will look at long multiplication and division.

Long multiplication

There are two popular methods for long multiplication: the traditional method and a method of boxes. Both rely on splitting numbers into their individual parts (hundreds, tens and units, etc.).

Traditional method
To calculate 456 × 78:

```
H  T  U    First line up the numbers into hundreds (H), tens (T)
4  5  6    and units (U).
×  7  8
_____
```

When using the traditional method, you multiply the number on the top row by the units and the tens separately, and then add the two results together.

First, multiply the numbers in the top row by the units (8), i.e. 8 × 6. Eight times six equals forty-eight. Write the 8 in the units column of the answer row and carry over the 4 to the tens column:

```
H  T  U
4  5  6
×  7  8
_____
      8
   4
```

Next, multiply by the next number in the top row, i.e. 8 × 5 which equals 40. Also add on the 4 that was carried over from the last step – this makes a total of 44. Write the 4 in the tens column and carry over the 4 to the hundreds column:

```
H  T  U
4  5  6
×  7  8
_____
   4  8
4  4
```

Next, multiply by the next number in the top row, i.e. 8 × 4 which equals 32. Also add on the 4 that was carried over from the last step – this makes a total of 36. Write down 36. You don't need to carry the 3, as there are no more numbers to multiply on this line:

```
Th H  T  U
    4  5  6
  × 7  8
3 6  4  8
    4  4
```

Now we have to multiply by the tens. First, add a zero on the right-hand side of the next answer row. This is because we want to multiply by 70 (7 tens), which is the same as multiplying by 10 and by 7:

```
Th H  T  U
    4  5  6
  × 7  8
3 6  4  8
          0
```

Multiply as before – this time it is 7 × 6, which equals 42. Place the 2 next to the zero and carry over the 4 to the hundreds column:

```
Th H  T  U
    4  5  6
  × 7  8
3 6  4  8
      2  0
   4
```

Next, multiply 7 × 5, which equals 35 and add on the 4 carried over to make a total of 39. Write down the 9 and carry over the 3:

```
Th H  T  U
    4  5  6
  × 7  8
3 6  4  8
      9  2  0
   3  4
```

Finally, multiply 7 × 4, which equals 28. Add the 3 to equal 31 and write down 31. You don't need to carry the 3, as there are no more numbers to multiply on this line:

```
  Th H  T  U
      4  5  6
    × 7  8
    3 6  4  8
  3 1  9  2  0
```

Now you're done with multiplying; you just need to add together 3,648 and 31,920. Write a plus sign to remind you of this:

```
     Th  H   T   U
          4   5   6
          ×   7   8
     ───────────────
      3   6   4   8
 +   3   1   9   2   0
     ───────────────
     3   5   5   6   8
          1
```

As before, carry over numbers (if necessary) when adding together.

You should get a final answer of 35,568.

When multiplying numbers with more than two digits, follow these steps: first multiply the top number by the units, then add a zero and multiply by the tens, then add two zeros and multiply by the hundreds, then add three zeros and multiply by the thousands, and so on. Add up all the resulting numbers at the end of each part answer.

Boxes method

In this method we split each number into its parts (thousands, hundreds, tens and units, etc.).

To calculate 456 × 78: 456 would be 400, 50 and 6:

	Th	H	T	U
456		400	50	6

78 would be 70 and 8.

	Th	H	T	U
78			70	8

We arrange these in a rectangle and multiply each part by the others. You need to be able to understand multiplying with powers of 10 to know how many zeros to put on the end of each part answer.

456 × 78			
	400	50	6
70	28 000	35 00	42 0
8	32 00	40 0	48

For the first sum, multiply 7 × 4 which equals 28. Now you need to add the zeros to ensure that the answer is of the right magnitude. Add three zeros (two from the 400 and one from the 70). Repeat for the other pairs.

We have worked out 400×70, 400×8, 50×70, 50×8, 6×70 and 6×8.

When this has all been done, you have to write out all the answers and add them together:

```
    2 8 0 0 0
        3 2 0 0
        3 5 0 0
          4 0 0
          4 2 0
+           4 8
    ─────────────
    3 5 5 6 8
    1 1
```

As before, carry over numbers (if necessary) when adding together.

You should get a final answer of 35,568.

Long division

As with multiplication, dividing large numbers can be daunting. But if the process is broken down into several steps, it is made a lot easier.

Before we start, a brief mention of the terms sometimes used might be useful. These are:

$$\frac{\text{dividend}}{\text{divisor}} = \text{quotient (answer)}$$

or

$$\text{divisor} \overline{\smash{)}\text{dividend}}^{\quad\text{quotient (answer)}}$$

The process is as follows.

WORKED EXAMPLE

Divide 3,612 by 14.

$$14 \overline{\smash{)}3\,6\,1\,2}$$

Firstly, divide the 14 into the first figure (i.e. the one on the left, which is 3). Obviously 14 into 3 will not go. So we then consider the next number (6) and ask how many times can 14 go into 36? Twice 14 equals 28; three times 14 equals 42. So, 14 goes into 36 2 times.

14 into 36 goes 2 times.
Multiply 2 × 14.
Subtract the 28 from 36.

$$14 \overline{)36 1 2} \begin{array}{r} 2 \\ \hline 3\ 6\ 1\ 2 \\ 2\ 8 \\ \hline 8 \end{array}$$

Bring down the next digit (1).

$$14 \overline{)3\ 6\ 1\ 2} \begin{array}{r} 2 \\ \hline 3\ 6\ 1\ 2 \\ 2\ 8 \downarrow \\ \hline 8\ 1 \end{array}$$

Then start the process again: divide 14 into 81. Once again, there is no exact number; 5 is the nearest (6 would be too much). If you are having trouble, a quicker method would be to write down the 14 times table before starting the division.

| 14 × 1 = 14 |
| 14 × 2 = 28 |
| 14 × 3 = 42 |
| 14 × 4 = 56 |
| 14 × 5 = 70 |
| 14 × 6 = 84 |
| 14 × 7 = 98 |
| 14 × 8 = 112 |
| 14 × 9 = 126 |
| 14 × 10 = 140 |

14 into 81 goes 5 times.
Multiply 14 × 5.
Subtract the 70 from 81.

$$14 \overline{)3\ 6\ 1\ 2} \begin{array}{r} 2\ 5 \\ \hline 3\ 6\ 1\ 2 \\ 2\ 8 \\ \hline 8\ 1 \\ 7\ 0 \\ \hline 1\ 1 \end{array}$$

Bring down the next digit (2)

$$14 \overline{)3\ 6\ 1\ 2} \begin{array}{r} 2\ 5 \\ \hline 3\ 6\ 1\ 2 \\ 2\ 8 \\ \hline 8\ 1 \\ 7\ 0 \downarrow \\ \hline 1\ 1\ 2 \end{array}$$

14 into 112 goes 8 times.
Multiply 14 × 8.
Subtract 112 − 11.

$$14 \overline{)3\ 6\ 1\ 2} \begin{array}{r} 2\ 5\ 8 \\ \hline 3\ 6\ 1\ 2 \\ 2\ 8 \\ \hline 8\ 1 \\ 7\ 0 \\ \hline 1\ 1\ 2 \\ 1\ 1\ 2 \\ \hline 0 \end{array}$$

Answer = 258

If there was a remainder at the end of the units then you would bring down a zero as the next number and place a decimal point in the answer.

WORKED EXAMPLE

23 divided by 17.

$$17\overline{)23}$$

Firstly, divide the 17 into the first figure (i.e. the one on the left, which is 2). Obviously 17 goes into 2 0 times or will not go. So we then consider the next number (3) and ask how many times can 17 go into 23? Obviously the answer is once; twice 17 equals 34. So, the answer is 1.

17 into 23 goes 1 time.
Multiply 1 × 17.
Subtract the 17 from 23.
So the answer is 1 remainder 6.

$$
\begin{array}{r}
1 \\
17\overline{)2\ 3} \\
\underline{1\ 7} \\
6
\end{array}
$$

This could also be expressed as $1\frac{6}{17}$, but we would usually calculate to 2 or more decimal places.

We can consider 23 being the same as 23.00000; therefore we can continue to divide the number:

$$
\begin{array}{r}
1. \\
17\overline{)2\ 3\ .\ 0} \\
\underline{1\ 7}\downarrow \\
60
\end{array}
$$

Bring down the zero and put decimal point in the answer.

Then start the process again:

| $17 \times 1 = 17$ |
| $17 \times 2 = 34$ |
| $17 \times 3 = 51$ |
| $17 \times 4 = 68$ |
| $17 \times 5 = 85$ |
| $17 \times 6 = 102$ |

17 into 60 goes 3 times.
Multiply 3 × 17.
Subtract the 51 from 60.
Bring down the next zero.

$$
\begin{array}{r}
1.3 \\
17\overline{)2\ 3\ .\ 0\ 0} \\
\underline{1\ 7} \\
60\downarrow \\
\underline{51} \\
9
\end{array}
$$

Repeat the process until there is no remainder or enough decimal places have been reached:

```
 17 × 1 = 17              1 . 3 5 2
 17 × 2  = 34        17 )2 3 . 0 0 0
 17 × 3 =  51           1 7
 17 × 4 = 68             6   0
 17 × 5 = 85             5   1
 17 × 6 = 102                9 0
                             8 5 ↓
       17 into 50 goes 2 times.        5 0
       Multiply 2 × 17.                 3 4
       Subtract the 34 from 50.         1 6
```

If we were working to 2 decimal places, our answer would be 1.35 (see 'Rounding of decimal numbers' later in the chapter).

Mathematical tricks and tips

An in-depth study of mathematics would reveal that certain patterns occur which can be used to our advantage to make calculations a lot easier. A few examples are given below.

Multiplication tips

Multiplying by 5

- Multiplying an **even** number by 5:
  - Halve the number you are multiplying and add a zero to give the answer. For example:

    5 × 8   Half of 8 is 4; add a zero for an answer of 40.

    5 × 1,234   Half of 1,234 is 617; add a zero for an answer of 6,170.

- Multiplying an **odd** number by 5:
  - Subtract one from the number you are multiplying, then halve that number and then place a 5 after the number to give you your answer. For example:

    5 × 7   Subtract 1 from the 7 (7 – 1) to get 6; halve the 6 to get 3, then place 5 after the number for an answer of 35.

    5 × 2,345   Subtract 1 from 2,345 (2,345 – 1) to get 2,344; halve that to get 1,172, then place 5 after the number for an answer of 11,725.

Note: all answers will end in 0 or 5.

Multiplying by 9

- Take the number you are multiplying and multiply by 10; then subtract the original number. For example:

    9 × 6   Multiply 6 by ten (6 × 10) which gives 60; subtract 6 from 60 (60 – 6) for an answer of 54.

9 × 1,234   Multiply 1,234 by ten (1,234 × 10) which gives 12,340; subtract 1,234 from 12,340 (12,340 − 1,234) for an answer of 11,106.

Note: adding up the digits of your answer together will equal 9 (not 11 × 9 = 99, but 9 + 9 = 18; 1 + 8 = 9) e.g.:

54   5 + 4 = 9

11,106   1 + 1+ 1 + 0 + 6 = 9

Multiplying by 11

- Multiplying by a single-digit number (i.e. up to 9): just "double" the number. For example:

    5 × 11   repeat the 5 for an answer of 55

    7 × 11   repeat the 7 for an answer of 77

- Multiplying a 2-digit number by 11: simply add the first and second digits and place the result between them. For example:

    36 × 11   3 + 6 = 9; place the 9 between the two digits (3 and 6) for an answer of 396.

    57 × 11   5 + 7 = 12; when the answer of the two digits is greater than 9, increase the left-hand number by 1 (i.e. carry over the 1):

                   5 _ 7 becomes 6 _ 7; insert the 2 (of the 12) in between the two digits for an answer of 627.

- Multiplying any number by 11: you add pairs of numbers together, except for those at each end – as you have to carry over 1 if the sum of the pairs is greater than 9, it makes it easier to work from right to left. For example:

324 × 11

- Write down the 4.
- Next add 4 and 2 (2 + 4 = 6). The answer is less than ten, so there is no number to carry over; write it down next to the 4, i.e. 64.
- Add 3 and 2 (2 + 3 = 5). The answer is less than ten, so there is no number to carry over; write it down next to the 64, i.e. 564.
- Write down the 3, i.e. 3564, for an answer of 3,564.

4,657 × 11

- Write down the 7.
- Next add 7 and 5 (7 + 5 = 12). The answer is greater than 9, so carry over 1; write down 2 next to the 7, i.e. 27.
- Add 6 and 5 (5 + 6 = 11); add the 1 carried over to give 12. Once again, the answer is greater than 9, so carry over 1; write down 2 next to the 27, i.e. 227.

- Add 6 and 4 (6 + 4 = 10), add the 1 carried over to give 11. Once again, the answer is greater than 9, so carry over 1; write down 1 next to the 227, i.e. 1,227.
- Add the 1 carried over to the last digit, i.e. 4 + 1 = 5.
- Write down 5 next to 1,227 for an answer of 51,227.

Multiplying by 16

- First, multiply the number you are multiplying by 10. Then halve the number and multiply by 10. Then add those two results together with the number itself to get your final answer.

For example: 16 × 28

- Step 1: Multiply the number by 10, i.e. 28 × 10 = 280.
- Step 2: Halve the number and multiply by 10, i.e. $\left(28 \times \frac{1}{2}\right) \times 10 = 14 \times 10 = 140$.
- Step 3: Add the results of steps 1 and 2 and the original number: 280 + 140 + 28 = 448

For example: 16 × 1,234

- Step 1: Multiply the number by 10, i.e. 1234 × 10 = 12,340.
- Step 2: Halve the number and multiply by 10, i.e. $\left(1,234 \times \frac{1}{2}\right) \times 10 = 617 \times 10 = 6,170$.
- Step 3: add the results of steps 1 and 2 and the original number: 12,340 + 6,170 + 1,234 = 19,744

Dividing tips

Dividing by 2

- All even numbers are divisible by 2, i.e. all numbers ending in 0, 2, 4, 6 or 8.
- Simply halve the number or divide by 2.

Dividing by 3

- Add up the digits: if the sum is divisible by 3, then the original number will be too. For example:

111,111   Add up the digits: 1 + 1 + 1 + 1 + 1 + 1 = 6; 6 can be divided by 3, so it follows that 111,111 can too: 111,111 ÷ 3 = 37,037.

87,676,896 Add up the digits: 8 + 7 + 6 + 7 + 6 + 8 + 9 + 6 = 57; then 5 + 7 = 12 which can be divided by 3, so it follows that 87,676,896 can too: 87, 676, 896 ÷ 3 = 29,225,632.

Dividing by 4

- If the last 2 digits of the number are divisible by 4, then the whole number is divisible by 4.
- An easy way of dividing is halving the number, then halving again.

For example:

259,812   The last two digits are 12 which is divisible by 4; so 259,812 is divisible by 4 as well.

$$259,812 \times \frac{1}{2} \times \frac{1}{2} = \frac{259,812}{4}$$

Half of 259,812 = 129,906; half of 129,906 = 64,953 to give an answer of 64,953.

Dividing by 5

• Numbers ending in a 5 or a 0 are always divisible by 5. For example:

12,345   Divide by 5 for an answer of 2,469.

Dividing by 6

• If the number is divisible by 3 and by 2, then it will be divisible by 6 as well.
  For example:

378   It is an even number so it is divisible by 2; 3 + 7 + 8 = 18, which is divisible by 3; so 378 will be divisible by 6: 378 ÷ 6 = 63.

120,540   It is an even number so it is divisible by 2; 1 + 2 + 0 + 5 + 4 + 0 = 12 which is divisible by 3; so 120,540 will be divisible by 6: 120, 540 ÷ 6 = 20,090.

Dividing by 7

• Take the last digit, double it, then subtract the answer from the remaining numbers; if that number is divisible by 7, then the original number is too. For example:

203   Take the last digit (3) and double it (2 × 3 = 6) to give 6. Subtract the 6 from the remaining numbers (20): 20 – 6 = 14. Is 14 divisible by 7? Yes, 14 ÷ 7 = 2; so 203 must be divisible by 7: 203 ÷ 7 = 29.

3,192   Take the last digit (2) and double it (2 × 2 = 4) to give 4. Subtract the 4 from the remaining numbers (319): 319 – 4 = 315. Is 315 divisible by 7? Yes, 315 ÷ 7 = 45; so 3,192 must be divisible by 7: 3,192 ÷ 7 = 456.

Dividing by 8

• If the last three digits are divisible by 8, so is the number. The three digit number (XYZ), will be divisible by 8 if: X is even and YZ are divisible by 8 or if X is odd and YZ – 4 is divisible by 8. For example:

2,360   Take the last three digits (XYZ = 360); the first digit (X = 3) is odd, so are the last two digits (YZ = 60) minus 4 divisible by 8? Yes, 60 − 4 = 56, 56 ÷ 8 = 7; so 2,360 must be divisible by 8: 2,360 ÷ 8 = 295.

65,184   Take the last three digits (XYZ = 184); the first digit (X = 1) is odd, so are the last two digits (YZ = 84) minus 4 divisible by 8? Yes, 84 − 4 = 80, 80 ÷ 8 = 10; so 65,184 must be divisible by 8: 65,184 ÷ 8 = 8,148.

424   This is a three digit number (XYZ = 424); the first digit (X = 4) is even, so are the last two digits (YZ = 24) divisible by 8? Yes, 24 ÷ 8 = 3; so 424 must be divisible by 8: 424 ÷ 8 = 53.

Dividing by 9

- If the sum of all the digits is divisible by 9, then the number will be too. **Note:** it will also be divisible by 3. For example:

270   Add up the digits: 2 + 7 + 0 = 9; 9 can be divided by 9, so it follows that 270 can too: 270 ÷ 9 = 30. NB: 270 ÷ 3 = 90.

641,232   Add up the digits: 6 + 4 + 1 + 2 + 3 + 2 = 18; 18 is divisible by 9, so it follows that 641,232 is as well: 641,232 ÷ 9 = 71,248. NB: 641,232 ÷ 3 = 213,744.

Dividing by 10

- Numbers ending in a 0 are always divisible by 10 (simply remove the zero at the end). For example:

7,890   Divide by 10: remove the zero for an answer of 789.

RULES OF ARITHMETIC

Now that we have covered basic multiplication and division, in what order should we perform an arithmetic sum?

Consider the sum: 3 + 4 × 6

- Do we add 3 and 4 together, and then multiply by 6, to give 42? *Or*
- Do we multiply 4 by 6, and then add 3, to give 27?

There are two possible answers depending upon how you solve the above sum – which one is right?

The correct answer is 27.

Rules for the order of operations

The processes of adding (+), subtracting (−), multiplying (×) and dividing (/ or ÷) numbers are known as **operations**. When you have complicated sums to do, you have to follow simple rules known as the **order of operations**. Initially (a long time ago) people agreed on an order in which mathematical operations should be performed, and this has been universally adopted.

The acronym or word **BEDMAS** is used to remember the correct order of operations: Each letter stands for a common mathematical operation; the **order** of the letter matches the **order** in which we do the mathematical operations.

B	stands for	'brackets'	e.g. (3 + 3)
E	stands for	'exponents' or 'exponentiation'	e.g. 2^3
D	stands for	'division'	e.g. 6 ÷ 3
M	stands for	'multiplication'	e.g. 3 × 4
A	stands for	'addition'	e.g. 3 + 4
S	stands for	'subtraction'	e.g. 4 – 3

TIP BOX

The basic rule is to work from **left** to **right**.

Consider the following simple sum: 10 – 3 + 2.
Remember – work from left to right.

10 – 3 = 7   then   7 + 2 = 9   9 is the right answer.

B	Calculations in **brackets** are done first. When you have more than one set of brackets, do the inner brackets first.
E	Next, any **exponentiation** (or powers) must be done – see later for a fuller explanation of exponentiation or powers.
D and **M**	Do the **division** and **multiplication** in order from left to right.
A and **S**	Do the **addition** and **subtraction** in order from left to right.

To help you to remember the rules, you can remember the acronym **BEDMAS** or the phrase Big Eaters Demand More Apple pie on Sundays. You can even make up your own phrase to remember the correct order of operations.

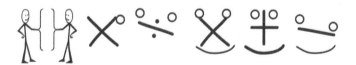

WORKED EXAMPLE

Work out the sum: $20 \div (12 - 2) \times 3^2 - 2$.

First of all – everything in brackets is done first:

$$(12 - 2) = 10$$

So the sum becomes:

$$20 \div 10 \times 3^2 - 2$$

Next, calculate the exponential:

$$3^2 = 3 \times 3 = 9$$

So the sum becomes:

$$20 \div 10 \times 9 - 2$$

Next multiply and divide as the operators appear:

$$20 \div 10 = 2$$

Then multiply:

$$2 \times 9 = 18$$

So the sum becomes:

$$18 - 2$$

Finally, add or subtract as the operators appear:

$$18 - 2 = 16$$

ANSWER: 16

TIP BOX

If there is a 'line', work out the top, then the bottom, and finally divide.

WORKED EXAMPLE

If we look at the example from Appendix 5 (calculating creatinine clearance), we can see that it is quite a complicated sum:

$$\text{CrCl (mL/min)} = \frac{1.23 \times (140 - 67) \times 72}{125} = 51.7$$

In the top line, do the sum within the brackets first, i.e. $(140 - 67)$, then multiply by 1.23 and then by 72.

Thus, $(140 - 67) = 73$, so the sum is $1.23 \times 73 \times 72 = 6,464.88$.

Then divide by 125 to give the answer of 51.7 (to one decimal place).

ANSWER: 51.7

FRACTIONS AND DECIMALS

A basic knowledge of fractions and decimals is helpful since they are involved in most calculations. It is important to know how to multiply and divide fractions and decimals, as well as to be able to convert from a fraction to a decimal and vice versa.

Fractions

Before we look at fractions, a few points need to be defined to make explanations easier.

Definition of a fraction

A fraction is part of a whole number or one number divided by another.

For example: $\frac{2}{5}$ is a fraction and means 2 parts of 5 (where 5 is the whole).

The number above the 'line' is called the **numerator**. It indicates the number of parts of the whole number that are being used (i.e. 2 in the above example).

The number below the 'line' is called the **denominator**. It indicates the number of parts into which the whole is divided (i.e. 5 in the above example).

Thus in the above example, the whole has been divided into 5 equal parts and you are dealing with 2 parts of the whole.

$$\frac{2 \quad \text{numerator}}{5 \quad \text{denominator}}$$

Simplifying (reducing) fractions

When you haven't got a calculator handy, it is often easier to work with fractions that have been 'simplified' or reduced to their lowest terms.

To reduce a fraction, choose any number that divides exactly into the numerator (number on the top) and the denominator (number on the bottom).

A fraction is said to have been reduced to its lowest terms when it is no longer possible to divide the numerator and denominator by the same number. This process of converting or reducing fractions to their simplest form is called **cancellation**. Remember: '*Whatever you do to the top line, you must do to the bottom line*'.

Remember – reducing or simplifying a fraction to its lowest terms does not change the value of the fraction.

WORKED EXAMPLES

1.
$$\frac{\cancel{15}}{\cancel{25}} = \frac{3}{5}$$

(showing 3 above 15, 5 below 25)

2.
$$\frac{\cancel{\cancel{135}}}{\cancel{\cancel{315}}} = \frac{3}{7}$$

(showing 3, 27 above 135; 63, 7 below 315)

15 and 25 are divided by 5.

a) 135 and 315 are divided by 5.
b) 27 and 63 are divided by 9.

Remember:

- Any number that ends in 0 or 5 is divisible by 5.
- Any even number is divisible by 2.
- There can be more than one step (see example 2 above).

If you have a calculator, then there is no need to reduce fractions to their lowest terms: the calculator does all the hard work for you!

Equivalent fractions

Consider the following fractions:

$$\frac{1}{2} \quad \frac{3}{6} \quad \frac{4}{8} \quad \frac{12}{24}$$

Each of the above fractions has the same value: they are called **equivalent** fractions.

If you reduce them to their simplest forms, you will notice that each is exactly a half.

Now consider the following fractions:

$$\frac{1}{3} \quad \frac{1}{4} \quad \frac{1}{6}$$

If you want to convert them to equivalent fractions with the **same** denominator, you have to find a common number that is divisible by all the individual denominators. For example, in the above case, multiply each denominator by 2, 3, 4, etc. until the smallest common number is found, as illustrated in the following table:

	3	4	6
×2	6	8	12
×3	9	12	18
×4	12	16	24

In this case, the common denominator is 12. For each fraction, multiply the numbers above and below the line by the common multiple. So for the first fraction, multiply the numbers above and below the line by 4; for the second multiply them by 3; and the third multiply them by 2. So the fractions become:

$$\frac{1}{3}\times\frac{4}{4}=\frac{4}{12} \text{ and } \frac{1}{3}\times\frac{3}{4}=\frac{3}{12} \text{ and } \frac{1}{6}\times\frac{2}{2}=\frac{2}{12}$$

$$\frac{1}{3}, \frac{1}{4} \text{ and } \frac{1}{6} \text{ equal } \frac{4}{12}, \frac{3}{12} \text{ and } \frac{2}{12}, \text{ respectively.}$$

Adding and subtracting fractions

To add (or subtract) fractions with the **same** denominator, add (or subtract) the numerators and place the result over the common denominator. For example:

$$\frac{14}{32}+\frac{7}{32}-\frac{4}{32}=\frac{14+7-4}{32}=\frac{17}{32}$$

To add (or subtract) fractions with the **different** denominators, first convert them to equivalent fractions with the same denominator, then add (or subtract) the numerators and place the result over the common denominator as before. For example:

$$\frac{1}{4}-\frac{1}{6}+\frac{1}{3}=\frac{3}{12}-\frac{2}{12}+\frac{4}{12}=\frac{3-2+4}{12}=\frac{5}{12}$$

Multiplying fractions

It is quite easy to multiply fractions. You simply multiply all the numbers 'above the line' (the numerators) together and then the numbers 'below the line' (the denominators). For example:

$$\frac{2}{5}\times\frac{3}{7}=\frac{2\times3}{5\times7}=\frac{6}{35}$$

However, it may be possible to 'simplify' the fraction before multiplying, e.g.

$$\frac{\overset{3}{\cancel{9}}}{\underset{5}{\cancel{15}}}\times\frac{2}{5}=\frac{3\times2}{5\times5}=\frac{6}{25}$$

In this case, the first fraction has first been reduced to its lowest terms by dividing both the numerator and denominator by 3.

You can sometimes 'reduce' both fractions by dividing diagonally by a common number, e.g.

$$\frac{\overset{2}{\cancel{6}}}{7}\times\frac{5}{\underset{3}{\cancel{9}}}=\frac{2\times5}{7\times3}=\frac{10}{21}$$

In this case, in both fractions there was a number that is divisible by 3 (6 and 9).

Dividing fractions

Sometimes it may be necessary to divide fractions. You will probably encounter fractions expressed or written like this:

$$\frac{\dfrac{2}{5}}{\dfrac{3}{7}} \text{ which is the same as } \frac{2}{5} \div \frac{3}{7}$$

In this case, you simply invert the second fraction (or the bottom one) and multiply, i.e.

$$\frac{2}{5} \div \frac{3}{7} = \frac{2}{5} \times \frac{7}{3} = \frac{2 \times 7}{5 \times 3} = \frac{14}{15}$$

If, after inverting, you see that reduction or cancellation is possible, you can do this before multiplying. For example:

$$\frac{5}{2} \div \frac{25}{8}$$

Cancelling diagonally, this becomes:

$$\frac{\overset{1}{\cancel{5}}}{\underset{1}{\cancel{2}}} \times \frac{\overset{4}{\cancel{8}}}{\underset{5}{\cancel{25}}} = \frac{1 \times 4}{1 \times 5} = \frac{4}{5}$$

TIP BOX

When doing any sum involving fractions, simplifying the fractions will make the calculation easier to do.

Converting fractions to decimals

This is quite easy to do. You simply divide the top number (numerator) by the bottom number (denominator).

If we use our original example:

$$\frac{2}{5} \text{ which can be re-written as } 2 \div 5 \text{ or } 5\overline{)2}$$

$$\begin{array}{r} 0.4 \\ 5\overline{)2.0} \\ \underline{2.0} \\ 0 \end{array}$$

It is important to place the decimal point in the correct position, usually after the number that is being divided (in this case 2).

Decimals

Decimals describe 'tenths' of a number, i.e. in terms of 10. A decimal number consists of a decimal point and numbers both to the left and right of that decimal point. Just as whole numbers have positions for units, tens, hundreds, etc., so do decimal numbers, but on **both** sides of the decimal point:

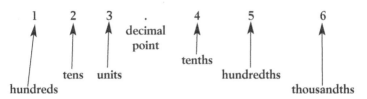

Numbers to the **left** of the **decimal point** are **greater than one.**
Numbers to the **right** of the **decimal point** are **less than one.**
Thus:

0.25 is a fraction of 1.

1.25 is 1 plus a fraction of 1.

Multiplying decimals

Decimals are multiplied in the same way as whole numbers except there is the decimal point to worry about.

If you are not using a calculator, don't forget to put the decimal point in the correct place in the answer.

Consider the sum: 0.65 × 0.75.

At first, it looks a bit daunting with the decimal points, but the principles covered earlier with long multiplication also apply here. You just have to be careful with the decimal point.

$$\begin{array}{r} 0\,.\,6\,5 \\ \times\ 0\,.\,7\,5 \\ \hline \end{array}$$

In essence, you are multiplying '65' by '75'

$$\begin{array}{r} 6\,5 \\ \times\ 7\,5 \\ \hline \end{array}$$

First, multiply the top row by 5:

$$\begin{array}{r} 6\,5 \\ \times\ 7\,5 \\ \hline 3\,2\,\underset{2}{2}\,5 \end{array}$$

Next, multiply the top row by 7 (don't forget to place a zero at the end of the second line):

$$\begin{array}{r} 6\,5 \\ \times\,7\,5 \\ \hline 3\,2\,5 \\ 4\,5\underset{3}{5}\,0 \end{array}$$

Now add the two lines together:

$$\begin{array}{r} 6\,5 \\ \times\,7\,5 \\ \hline 3\,2\,5 \\ 4\,5\,5\,0 \\ \hline 4\,8\,7\,5 \end{array}$$

Finally, we have to decide where to place the decimal point.

The decimal point is placed as many places to the **left** as there are numbers after it in the sum. In this case there are four;

$$0\,.\,6\,5\ \times\ 0\,.\,7\,5$$
$$1\ 23\ 4$$

Therefore in the answer, the decimal point is put 4 places to the **left**.

$$\overset{\frown}{.4\ 8\ 7\ 5} = 0.4875$$

Multiplying by multiples of 10

To multiply a decimal by multiples of 10 (100, 1,000, etc.) you simply move the decimal point as many places to the *right* as there are zeros in the number you are multiplying by. For example:

MULTIPLY TO BY	NUMBER OF ZEROS	MOVE THE DECIMAL POINT TO THE RIGHT
10	1	1 place
100	2	2 places
1,000	3	3 places
10,000	4	4 places

For example:

$$546 \times 1,000$$

Move the decimal point THREE places to the RIGHT. (There are THREE zeros in the number it is being multiplied by.)

$$5 \quad 4 \quad 6 \overset{\frown}{.} 0 \quad 0 \quad 0 = 546{,}000$$

Dividing decimals

Once again, decimals are divided in the same way as whole numbers except there is a decimal point to worry about.

A recap of the terms sometimes used might be useful. These are:

$$\frac{\text{dividend}}{\text{divisor}} = \text{quotient (answer)}$$

or

$$\text{divisor} \overline{\left) \text{dividend} \right.} \quad \overset{\text{quotient (answer)}}{}$$

WORKED EXAMPLE

Consider $\frac{34.8}{4}$ which can be re-written as $34.8 \div 4$ or $4\overline{\smash{\big)}3\ 4\ .\ 8}$.

The decimal point in the answer (quotient) is placed directly above the decimal point in the dividend:

$$4\overline{\smash{\big)}3\ 4\ \overset{.}{.}\ 8}$$

Firstly, divide the 4 into the first figure (i.e. the one on the left, which is 3). Obviously dividing 4 into 3 goes 0 times or will not go. So we then consider the next number (4) and ask how many times can 4 go into 34? Eight times 4 equals 32; nine times 4 equals 36. So, the answer is 8.

Divide 4 into 34, it goes 8 times.

Multiply 4 × 8.
Subtract 32 from 34.
Bring down the next number (8).

$$\begin{array}{r} 8 \\ 4\overline{\smash{\big)}3\ 4\ .\ 8} \\ 3\ 2\downarrow \\ \hline 2\ 8 \end{array}$$

Place the decimal point in the answer (quotient) above the point in the dividend. Then start the process again:

$$\begin{array}{r} 8\ .\ 7 \\ 4\overline{\smash{\big)}3\ 4\ .\ 8} \\ 3\ 2 \\ \hline 2\ \ 8 \\ 2\ \ 8 \\ \hline 0 \end{array}$$

4 into 28 goes 7 times.
Multiply 4 × 7.
Subtract 28 from 28.

What do we do when both the divisor and dividend are decimals?

WORKED EXAMPLE

Consider $\dfrac{1.55}{0.2}$ which can be re-written as $1.55 \div 0.2$ or $0.2 \overline{)1.55}$.

- First make the **divisor** a **whole number**, i.e. in this case, move the decimal point **one** place to the **right.**
- Then, move the decimal point in the **dividend** the **same number** of places to the **right.**

In this case:

$$0.2 \qquad 1.55$$

Now the division is:

$$2 \overline{)15.5}$$

The decimal point in the answer (quotient) is placed directly above the decimal point in the dividend:

$$2 \overline{)15.5}$$

Perform the same steps as for the example previous:

2 into 15 goes 7 times.
Multiply 2×7.
Subtract 14 from 15.

$$\begin{array}{r} 7 \\ 2 \overline{)15.5} \\ 14 \\ \hline 1 \end{array}$$

Bring down the next number (5).

$$\begin{array}{r} 7 \\ 2 \overline{)15.5} \\ 14 \downarrow \\ \hline 1\ \ 5 \end{array}$$

2 into 15 goes 7 times.
Multiply 2×7.
Subtract 14 from 15.

$$\begin{array}{r} 7.7 \\ 2 \overline{)15.5} \\ 14 \\ \hline 1\ \ 5 \\ 1\ \ 4 \\ \hline 1 \end{array}$$

Place the decimal point in the answer (quotient) above the point in the dividend

$$
\begin{array}{r}
7\ .\ 7 \\
2\,\overline{)\,1\ 5\ .\ 5\ 0} \\
\underline{1\ 4} \\
1\ \ 5 \\
\underline{1\ \ 4} \\
1\ \ 0
\end{array}
$$

Bring down a zero (0).

Repeat as before:

$$
\begin{array}{r}
7\ .\ 7\ 5 \\
2\,\overline{)\,1\ 5\ .\ 5\ 0} \\
\underline{1\ 4} \\
1\ \ 5 \\
\underline{1\ \ 4} \\
1\ \ 0 \\
\underline{1\ \ 0} \\
0
\end{array}
$$

2 into 10 goes 5 times.
Multiply 2×5.
Subtract 10 from 10.

ANSWER: So the answer is 7.75.

Dividing by multiples of 10

To divide a decimal by a multiple of 10, you simply move the decimal point the same number of places to the LEFT as there are zeros in the number you are dividing by. For example:

NUMBER TO DIVIDE BY	NUMBER OF ZEROS	MOVE THE DECIMAL POINT TO THE LEFT
10	1	1 place
100	2	2 places
1,000	3	3 places
10,000	4	4 places

For example:

$$
\frac{546}{1{,}000}
$$

Move the decimal point three places to the left. (There are three zeros in the bottom number, the divisior.)

$$
0\ .\ 5\ \ 4\ \ 6
$$

Rounding of decimal numbers

Sometimes it is necessary to 'round up' or 'round down' a decimal number to a whole number. This is particularly true in infusion rate calculations, as it is impossible to give a part of a drop or a millilitre (mL) when setting an infusion rate.

If the number after the decimal point is 4 or less, then ignore it, i.e. 'round down'.

For example: 31.25: The number after the decimal point is 2 (which is less than 4), so it rounds down to 31.

If the number after the decimal point is 5 or more, then add 1 to the whole number, i.e. 'round up'.

For example: 41.67: The number after the decimal point is 6 (which is more than 5), so it rounds up to 42.

Converting decimals to fractions

It is unlikely that you would want to convert a decimal to a fraction in any calculation, but this is included here just in case.

- First you have to make the decimal a whole number by moving the decimal point to the RIGHT, e.g.

$$0.75 \quad \text{becomes} \quad 75 \quad \text{(the \textbf{numerator} in the fraction)}$$

- Next divide by a multiple of 10 (the **denominator**) to make a fraction. The value of this multiple of 10 is determined by how many places to the **right** the decimal point has moved, i.e.

1 place = a denominator of 10
2 places = a denominator of 100
3 places = a denominator of 1,000

Thus in our example 0.75 becomes 75, i.e. the decimal point has moved 2 places to the right, so the denominator will be 100:

$$0.75 = \frac{75}{100}$$

To simplify this fraction, divide both the numerator and denominator by 25:

$$0.75 = \frac{75}{100} = \frac{3}{4}$$

ROMAN NUMERALS

Although it is not recommended as best practice, Roman numerals are still commonly used when writing prescriptions. In Roman numerals, letters are used to designate numbers.

The following table explains the Roman numerals most commonly seen on prescriptions.

ROMAN NUMERAL	ORDINARY NUMBER
I (or i)	1
II (or ii)	2
III (or iii)	3
IV (or iv)	4
V (or v)	5
VI (or vi)	6
VII (or vii)	7
VIII (or viii)	8
IX (or ix)	9
X (or x)	10
L (or l)	50
C (or c)	100
D (or d)	500
M (or m)	1,000

Rules for reading Roman numerals

There are some simple rules for reading Roman numerals. It doesn't matter whether they are capital letters or small letters, the value is the same. The position of one letter relative to another is very important and determines the value of the numeral.

- **Rule 1**: Repeating a Roman numeral twice doubles its value; repeating it three times triples its value, e.g.

$$II = (I + I) = 2; III = (I + I + I) = 3$$

- **Rule 2**: The letter I can usually be repeated up to three times; the letter V is written **once** only, e.g.

$$III = 3 \text{ is correct; } IIII = 4 \text{ is not correct}$$

- **Rule 3**: When a smaller Roman numeral is placed **after** a larger one, **add** the two together, e.g.

$$VI = 5 + I = 6$$

- **Rule 4**: When a smaller Roman numeral is placed **before** a larger one, **subtract** the smaller numeral from the larger one, e.g.

$$IV = 5 - I = 4$$

- **Rule 5**: When a Roman numeral of a smaller value comes between two of larger values, first apply the subtraction rule, then add, e.g.

$$XIV = 10 + (5 - I) = 10 + 4 = 14$$

POWERS OR EXPONENTIALS

Powers or exponentials are a convenient way of writing very large or very small numbers. Powers of 10 are often used in scientific calculations.

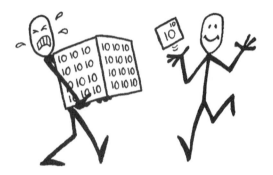

Consider the following:

$$10 \times 10 \times 10 \times 10 \times 10$$

Here you are multiplying by 10, five times. Instead of all these 10s, you can write:

$$10^5$$

We say this as '10 to the power of 5' or just '10 to the 5'. The small raised number 5 next to the 10 is known as the **power** or **exponent** – it tells you how many of the same number are being multiplied together.

$$10^5 \diagdown \text{ power or exponent}$$

We came across the terms 'exponent' or 'exponentiation' when looking at the rules of arithmetic earlier. Now consider this:

$$\frac{1}{10} \times \frac{1}{10} \times \frac{1}{10} \times \frac{1}{10} \times \frac{1}{10} = \frac{1}{10 \times 10 \times 10 \times 10 \times 10}$$

Here we are repeatedly dividing by 10. For short you can write:

$$10^{-5} \text{ instead of } \frac{1}{10 \times 10 \times 10 \times 10 \times 10}$$

In this case, you will notice that there is a minus sign next to the power or exponent.

$$10^{-5} \diagdown \text{ minus power or exponent}$$

This is a **negative power** or **exponent**, and is usually read '10 to the power of –5' or just '10 to the minus 5'.

In conclusion:

- A positive power or exponent means **multiply** the base number by itself the number of times of the power or exponent;
- A negative power or exponent means **divide** the base number by itself the number of times of the power or exponent.

You will probably come across powers used in the following way:

$$3 \times 10^3 \text{ or } 5 \times 10^{-2}$$

This is known as the **standard index form**. It is a combination of a power of 10 and a number with one unit in front of a decimal point, e.g.

$$5 \times 10^6 \qquad (5.0 \times 10^6)$$
$$1.2 \times 10^3$$
$$4.5 \times 10^{-2}$$
$$3 \times 10^{-6} \qquad (3.0 \times 10^{-6})$$

The number in front of decimal point can be anything from 0 to 9.

This type of notation is seen on a scientific calculator when you are working with very large or very small numbers. It is a common and convenient way of describing numbers without having to write a lot of zeros.

Here are some more examples:

$$3 \times 10^5 \qquad = 3 \times 100,000 \qquad = 300,000$$
$$1.4 \times 10^3 \qquad = 1.4 \times 1,000 \qquad = 1,400$$
$$4 \times 10^{-2} \qquad = 4 \div 100 \qquad = 0.04$$
$$2.25 \times 10^{-3} \qquad = 2.25 \div 1,000 \qquad = 0.00225$$

Because you are dealing in 10s, you will notice that the 'number of noughts' you multiply or divide by is equal to the power. For example:

I. 3×10^5 You move the decimal point **five** places to the **right** (positive power of 5)

So it becomes:

$$3 \times 10^5 = \underbrace{3\,0\,0\,0\,0\,0\,.}_{5 \text{ noughts}} = 300,000$$

2. 4×10^{-2} You move the decimal point **two** places to the **left** (negative power of 2)

So it becomes:

$$4 \times 10^{-2} = \underbrace{0\,.\,0\,4}_{2 \text{ noughts}} = 0.04$$

The table below summarizes the commonly used powers of 10 and their equivalent numbers

POWER OF TEN	STANDARD FORM
10^9	1,000,000,000
10^8	100,000,000
10^7	10,000,000
10^6	1,000,000
10^5	100,000
10^4	10,000
10^3	1,000
10^2	100
10^1	10
10^0	1
10^{-1}	0.1
10^{-2}	0.01
10^{-3}	0.001
10^{-4}	0.0001
10^{-5}	0.00001
10^{-6}	0.000001
10^{-7}	0.0000001
10^{-8}	0.00000001
10^{-9}	0.000000001

USING A CALCULATOR

Numbers should be entered in a certain way when using a calculator, and you need to know how to read the display. The manual or instructions that came with your calculator will tell you how to do this.

This section will help you to learn how to use your calculator properly. Just follow the rules of arithmetic which we covered earlier.

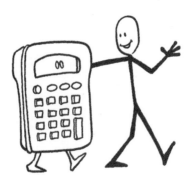

Consider the following:

$$\frac{2}{500} \times 140$$

There are two ways of entering this into your calculator:

Method 1

Enter [2]	DISPLAY = 2
Enter [×]	DISPLAY = 2
Enter [1][4][0]	DISPLAY = 140

You are doing the sum: 2×140

Enter [÷]	DISPLAY = 280
Enter [5][0][0]	DISPLAY = 500

You are now doing the sum: $\dfrac{2 \times 140}{500}$

Enter [=]	DISPLAY = 0.56 (answer)

Method 2

Enter [2]	DISPLAY = 2
Enter [÷]	DISPLAY = 2
Enter [5][0][0]	DISPLAY = 500

You are doing the sum: $\dfrac{2}{500}$

Enter [×]	DISPLAY = 4^{-03} or 0.004

This is the way a scientific calculator shows small numbers (see section on 'Powers or exponentials').

Enter [1][4][0]   DISPLAY = 140

You are doing the sum: $\dfrac{2}{500} \times 140$

Enter [=]   DISPLAY = 0.56 (answer)

Now consider the following sum:

$$\frac{20}{60} \times \frac{1,000}{8}$$

Again, there are two possible ways of doing this:

Method 1

Enter [2][0]   DISPLAY = 20
Enter [÷]   DISPLAY = 20
Enter [6][0]   DISPLAY = 60

You are doing the sum: $\dfrac{20}{60}$

Enter [×]   DISPLAY = 0.3333333
Enter [1][0][0][0]   DISPLAY = 1000

You are doing the sum: $\dfrac{20}{60} \times 1,000$

Enter [÷]   DISPLAY = 333.33333
Enter [8]   DISPLAY = 8

You are doing the sum: $\dfrac{20}{60} \times \dfrac{1,000}{8}$

Enter [=]   DISPLAY = 41.66667 (answer)

Method 2

Enter [2][0]   DISPLAY = 20
Enter [×]   DISPLAY = 20
Enter [1][0][0][0]   DISPLAY = 1000

You are doing the sum: 20 × 1,000

Enter [÷]   DISPLAY = 20000
Enter [6][0]   DISPLAY = 60

You are doing the sum: $\dfrac{20 \times 1,000}{60}$

Enter [÷]   DISPLAY = 333.33333
Enter [8]   DISPLAY = 8

You are doing the sum: $\dfrac{20 \times 1,000}{60 \times 8}$

Enter [=]   DISPLAY = 41.66667 (answer)

Whichever method you use, the answer is the same. However, it may be easier to split the sum into two parts, i.e.

$$20 \times 1,000 \quad (1)$$

and

$$60 \times 8 \quad (2)$$

Then divide (1) by (2), i.e.

$$\frac{20}{60} \times \frac{1,000}{8} = \frac{20,000}{480} = 41.6667$$

Now consider this sum:

$$\frac{6}{4 \times 5}$$

You can either simplify the sum, i.e. $\dfrac{6}{20}$, then divide 6 by 20 = 0.3 (answer).

Alternatively, you could enter the following on your calculator:

Enter [6]   DISPLAY = 6
Enter [÷]   DISPLAY = 6
Enter [4]   DISPLAY = 4

You are doing the sum: $\dfrac{6}{4} = 1.5$

Enter [÷]   DISPLAY = 1.5
Enter [5]   DISPLAY = 5

You are doing the sum: $\dfrac{\frac{6}{4}}{5}$ i.e. $\dfrac{1.5}{5}$

Enter [=]   DISPLAY = 0.3 (answer)

Again, you can use either method, but it may be easier to simplify the top line and the bottom line before dividing the two.

See the section on 'Powers and calculators' for an explanation of how your calculator displays very large and small numbers.

TIP BOX

Get to know how to use your calculator – read the manual! If you don't know how to use your calculator properly, then there is always the potential for errors. You won't know if the answer you've got is correct or not.

POWERS AND CALCULATORS

The display on a normal calculator is usually eight numbers:

$$1\ 2\ 3\ 4\ 5\ 6\ 7\ 8$$

The maximum number that can be displayed in this way is therefore:

$$99,999,999$$

The smallest number that can be displayed is therefore:

$$0.0000001$$

On a scientific calculator, if an answer is either larger or smaller than that which can normally be displayed, then the answer will be shown as a power or exponential of 10. For example.

$$5.0^6 \ or \ 3.^{-06}$$

As mentioned earlier, this is known as **standard index form**.

$$5.0^6 = 5 \times 10^6 = 5 \times 1,000,000 = 5,000,000$$

$$3.^{-06} = 3 \times 10^{-6} = \frac{3}{1,000,000} = 0.000003$$

So if the answer is displayed like this on your calculator and you want to convert to an ordinary number, you simply move the decimal point the number of places indicated by the power, to the left or to the right depending on whether it is a negative or positive power. Looking at the same examples again:

$$5.0^6 = 5 \times 10^6 = \underbrace{5\,000000.}_{6\ zeros} = 5,000,000$$

$$3.^{-06} = 3 \times 10^{-6} = \underbrace{0.000003}_{6\ zeros} = 0.000003$$

ESTIMATING ANSWERS

It is often useful to be able to estimate the answer for a calculation. The estimating process is quite simple: numbers are either rounded up or down in terms of tens, hundreds or thousands to give numbers that can be calculated more easily.

For example, to the nearest ten, 41 would be rounded down to 40; 23.5 to 20; and 58.75 rounded up to 60. Single-digit numbers should be left as they are (although 8 and 9 could be rounded up to 10).

Once the numbers have been rounded up or down, it's possible to do a simple calculation, and the result is close enough to act as an estimate.

No set rules for estimating can be given to cover all the possibilities that may be encountered. The following examples should illustrate the principles involved. Don't forget – the answer is only an estimate.

- If you round numbers up, the estimated answer will be more than the actual answer.
- If you round numbers down, the estimated answer will be less than the actual answer.

WORKED EXAMPLE

Add the following numbers:

$$3,459 + 11,723 + 7,895 + 789$$

There are several methods for estimating the answer; you should pick the method most suited to you.

METHOD 1

- Change the numbers so that they can be easily added up in your head. Look at the numbers. Three are numbers in the thousands and one is in the hundreds. For now, ignore the number in the hundreds.
- First, add the thousands column (the numbers that are to the left of the comma), i.e.:

$$3 + 11 + 7 = 21$$

Then add three noughts (to convert back to a number in the thousands):

$$21,000$$

- Second, look at the hundreds column (the first numbers to the right of the comma in the numbers that are in the thousands). Add those numbers:

$$3,\underline{4}59 + 11,\underline{7}23 + 7,\underline{8}95 + \underline{7}89$$
$$4 \quad + \quad 7 \quad + \quad 8 \quad + 7 \ = 26$$

Then add two noughts (to convert back to a number in the hundreds):

$$2600 \ (2,600)$$

Round up or down to a number in the thousands (i.e. 3,000) and add to the 21,000:

$$21,000 + 3,000 = 24,000 \ \textit{Estimated answer}$$
$$3,459 + 11,723 + 7,895 + 789 = 23,866 \ \textit{Actual answer}$$

METHOD 2

Round the numbers up or down to numbers that can be added up easily. In this case:

NUMBER	NUMBER ROUNDED UP OR DOWN
3,459	3,500
11,723	11,700
7,895	7,900
789	800
23,866 *Actual answer*	23,900 *Estimated answer*

WORKED EXAMPLE

Multiply 3018 by 489.

STEP ONE

Round the numbers up or down to the nearest thousand or hundred, i.e.:

$$3018 \approx 3000 \text{ and } 489 \approx 500$$

You are now considering the sum 3000×500.

STEP TWO

For now, ignore the zeros in the sum, so consider the sum as:

$$3 \times 5 = 15$$

STEP THREE

Now bring back the zeros to ensure that the answer is of the right magnitude.

In this case 5 zeros were ignored, so add them to the end of the answer from Step Two:

$$15\ 00000 = 1,500,000$$

The estimated answer is 1,500,000.

The actual answer of the sum 3018×489 is 1,475,802.

WORKED EXAMPLE

Multiply 28.67 by 67.66.

STEP ONE

Round the numbers up or down to the nearest ten, i.e.:

$$28.85 \approx 30 \text{ and } 67.25 \approx 70$$

You are now considering the sum 30×70.

STEP TWO
For now, ignore the zeros in the sum, so consider the sum as

$$3 \times 7 = 21$$

STEP THREE
Now bring back the zeros to ensure that the answer is of the right magnitude.

In this case 2 zeros were ignored, so add them to the end of the answer from Step Two:

$$21\ 00 = 2,100$$

The estimated answer is 2,100.

The actual answer of the sum 28.85×67.25 is 1,940.1625.

REMEMBER

Don't forget – the answer is only an estimate.

If you **round up** numbers, the estimated answer will be **more** than the actual answer.

If you **round down** numbers, the estimated answer will be **less** than the actual answer

---

WORKED EXAMPLE

Divide 36,042 by 48.

STEP ONE
Round the numbers up or down in terms of thousands, hundreds and tens, i.e.

$$36,042 \approx 36,000 \text{ and } 48 \approx 50$$

You are now considering the sum $36,000 \div 50$.

STEP TWO
In division, more care is needed with the zeros. If there is a zero in the divisor (the number you are dividing by), then this must be cancelled out with a zero from the dividend (the number you are dividing). This may, at first, appear confusing, but the following may make it clearer:

$3\,6,0\,0\,\cancel{0} \div 5\,\cancel{0}$ Cancel out 1 zero from each side of the division sign ($\div$) to give 3,600 ÷ 5.

If there were two zeros in the divisor, then two zeros would have to be cancelled from the dividend, i.e.

$3\,6,0\,\cancel{0}\,\cancel{0} \div 5\,\cancel{0}\,\cancel{0}$ Cancel out 2 zeros from each side of the division sign ($\div$) to give 360 ÷ 5.

STEP THREE

For now the zeros in the sum can be ignored, so consider the sum as:

$$36 \div 5 = 7.2 \text{ (round down to 7)}$$

STEP FOUR

Now bring back the zeros to ensure that the answer is of the right magnitude. In this case two zeros were ignored, so add them to the end of the answer from Step Three:

$$7\ 00 = 700$$

The estimated answer is 700.

The actual answer of the sum 36,042 ÷ 48 is 750.875.

REMEMBER

The answer is only an estimate.

If you **round up** numbers, the estimated answer will be **more** than the actual answer.

If you **round down** numbers, the estimated answer will be **less** than the actual answer.

Numbers less than one

What happens if there is a number less than 1? You obviously cannot round down to zero, as this would not give a proper answer – multiplying anything by zero gives an answer of zero. You simply convert the number to a fraction (see the section on 'Converting decimals to fractions' on page 34).

If there is more than one number after the decimal point, then round up or down to one decimal place. For example

$$0.28 \text{ becomes } 0.3$$

Then convert to a fraction:

$$0.3 = \frac{3}{10}$$

TIP BOX

In this case, to convert to a fraction, *always* divide by 10.

Once the decimal has been converted to a fraction, calculate the sum as if you are multiplying or dividing by fractions (see the sections on 'Multiplying fractions and 'Dividing fractions' earlier). For example:

27×0.28	would become	$30 \times \dfrac{3}{10}$	(27 rounded up to 30)
$\dfrac{3}{\cancel{30}} \times \dfrac{3}{\cancel{10}}$	would become	$3 \times 3 = 9$	*Estimated answer*
27×0.28	$= 7.56$		*Actual answer*

OBJECTIVES

At the end of this chapter, you should be familiar with the following:
- Percent and percentages
- Converting fractions to percentages and vice versa
- Converting decimals to percentages and vice versa
- Calculations involving percentages
  - How to find the percentage of a number
  - How to find what percentage one number is of another
- Drug calculations involving percentages
- How to use the percentage key on your calculator

KEY POINTS

Per Cent
- Per cent means 'parts of a hundred' or a 'proportion of a hundred'.
- The symbol for per cent is %, so 30% means 30 parts or units of a hundred.
- Per centages are often used to give a quick indication of a specific quantity and are very useful when making comparisons.

Percentages and Fractions
- To convert a **fraction** to a **percentage**, **multiply** by 100.
- To convert a **percentage** to a **fraction**, **divide** by 100.

Percentages and Decimals
- To convert a **decimal** to a **percentage**, **multiply** by 100 – move the decimal point **two** places to the **right**.
- To convert a **percentage** to a **decimal**, **divide** by 100 – move the decimal point **two** places to the **left**.

Thus:

$$25\% = \frac{25}{100} = \frac{1}{4} = 0.25 \text{ (a quarter)}$$

$$33\% = \frac{33}{100} = \frac{1}{3} = 0.33 \text{ (approx. a third)}$$

$$50\% = \frac{50}{100} = \frac{1}{2} = 0.5 \text{ (a half)}$$

$$66\% = \frac{66}{100} = \frac{2}{3} = 0.66 \text{ (approx. two-thirds)}$$

$$75\% = \frac{75}{100} = \frac{3}{4} = 0.75 \text{ (three-quarters)}$$

To find the percentage of a number, always **divide** by 100:
$$\frac{\text{base}}{100} \times \text{per cent}$$
To find what percentage one number is of another, always **multiply** by 100:
$$\frac{\text{amount}}{\text{base}} \times 100$$

INTRODUCTION

The per cent or percentage is a common way of expressing the amount of something, and is very useful for comparing different quantities.

It is unlikely that you will need to calculate the percentage of something on the ward. It is more likely that you will need to know how much drug is in a solution given as a percentage, e.g. an infusion containing potassium 0.3%.

PER CENT AND PERCENTAGES

As stated before, a convenient way of expressing drug strengths is by using the per cent. We will be dealing with how percentages are used to describe drug strengths or concentrations in Chapter 5, 'Drug strengths or concentrations'.

The aim of this chapter is to explain the concept of per cent and how to do simple percentage calculations. It is important to understand per cent before moving on to percentage concentrations.

Per cent means 'parts of a hundred' or a 'proportion of a hundred' and the symbol for per cent is %. So 30 per cent (30%) means 30 parts or units of a hundred.

Percentages are often used to give a quick indication of a specific quantity and are very useful when making comparisons. If you consider a town where 5,690 people live and the unemployment number is 853, it is very difficult to visualize exactly how many or what proportion of the people are unemployed. It is much easier to say that in a town of 5,690 people, 15 per cent of them are unemployed.

If we consider another town of 11,230 people where 2,246 people are unemployed, it is very difficult, at a glance, to see which town has the greater proportion of unemployed. But when the numbers are given as percentages, it is much easier to compare: the first town has 15 per cent unemployment, whereas the second town has 20 per cent unemployed.

Percentages can be very useful, and so is being able to convert a number to a percentage. It is easier to compare numbers or quantities when they are given as percentages.

CONVERTING FRACTIONS TO PERCENTAGES
AND VICE VERSA

To convert a fraction to a percentage, you simply **multiply** by 100, e.g.

$$\frac{2}{5} = \left(\frac{2}{5} \times 100\right)\% = 40\%$$

Conversely, to convert a percentage to a fraction, **divide** by 100, i.e.

$$40\% = \frac{40}{100} = \frac{4}{10} = \frac{2}{5}$$

If possible, always reduce the fraction to its lowest terms before making the conversion.

CONVERTING DECIMALS TO PERCENTAGES
AND VICE VERSA

To convert a decimal to a percentage, once again you simply **multiply** by 100, e.g.

$$0.4 = \left(0.4 \times 100\right)\% = 40\%$$

Remember, to multiply by 100, you move the decimal point **two** places to the **right**.

To convert a percentage to a decimal, you **divide** by 100, e.g.

$$40\% = \frac{40}{100} = 0.4$$

Remember, to divide by 100, you move the decimal point **two** places to the **left**.

So, to convert fractions and decimals to percentages or vice versa, you simply multiply or divide by 100. Thus:

$$25\% = \frac{25}{100} = \frac{1}{4} = 0.25 \text{ (a quarter)}$$

$$33\% = \frac{33}{100} = \frac{1}{3} = 0.33 \text{ (approx. a third)}$$

$$50\% = \frac{50}{100} = \frac{1}{2} = 0.5 \text{ (a half)}$$

$$66\% = \frac{66}{100} = \frac{2}{3} = 0.66 \text{ (approx. two-thirds)}$$

$$75\% = \frac{75}{100} = \frac{3}{4} = 0.75 \text{ (three-quarters)}$$

The next step is to look at how to find the percentage of an amount. The Worked Example on the next page shows how this is done.

CALCULATIONS INVOLVING PERCENTAGES

The first type of calculation we are going to look at is how to find the percentage of a given quantity or number.

> **WORKED EXAMPLE**
> How much is 28% of 250?
> There are several ways of solving this type of problem.
>
> *METHOD 1: WORKING IN PERCENTAGES*
> With this method you are working in percentages.
>
> *STEP ONE*
> When doing percentage calculations, the number or quantity you want to find the percentage of, is always equal to 100%.
>   In this example, 250 is equal to 100% and you want to find out how much 28% is. So:
>
> $$250 = 100\%$$
>
> (Thus you are converting the number to a percentage.)
>
> *STEP TWO*
> Calculate how much is equal to 1%, i.e. divide by 100 (you are using the 'ONE unit' rule – see Chapter 1 'First principles' for an explanation):
>
> $$1\% = \frac{250}{100}$$
>
> *STEP THREE*
> Multiply by the percentage required (28%):
>
> $$28\% = \frac{250}{100} \times 28 = 70$$
>
> *ANSWER:* 28% of 250 is 70.
>
> *METHOD 2: WORKING IN FRACTIONS*
> In this method you are trying to find the fraction of the whole.
>
> *STEP ONE*
> First convert the percentage to a fraction, i.e. divide by 100:
>
> $$28\% = \frac{28}{100}$$

STEP TWO
Multiply by the original number (250) to find how much the fraction is of the whole:

$$\frac{28}{100} \times 250 = 70$$

Thus you are finding out how much the fraction is of the original number.

ANSWER: 28% of 250 is 70.

In both methods used, it can be seen that the number is always divided by 100; thus a simple formula can be devised. If we call the original number **base**; the amount we want to find out (i.e. the answer) the **amount**; and the percentage required, **per cent**, then we can write this as formula:

$$\text{amount} = \frac{\text{base}}{100} \times \text{per cent}$$

In this example:

$$\text{base} = 250$$
$$\text{per cent} = 28\%$$

Substituting the numbers in the formula:

$$\frac{250}{100} \times 28 = 70$$

ANSWER: 28% of 250 is 70.

TIP BOX

Whatever method you use, you always **divide** by 100.

However, you may want to find out what percentage a number is of another larger number, especially when comparing numbers or quantities. This is the second type of percentage calculation we are going to look at.

WORKED EXAMPLE
What percentage is 630 of 9,000?
In this case, it is best to work in percentages since that is what you want to find.

STEP ONE

Once again, the number or quantity you want to find the percentage of is always equal to 100%.

In this example, 9,000 would be equal to 100% and you want to find out the percentage that is 630. So:

$$9,000 = 100\%$$

(Thus you are converting the number to a percentage.)

STEP TWO

Calculate the percentage that is 1, i.e. divide by 9,000 using the 'ONE unit' rule:

$$1 = \frac{100}{9,000}\%$$

STEP THREE

Multiply by the number you wish to find the percentage of, i.e. the smaller number (630):

$$\frac{100}{9,000} \times 630 = 7\%$$

ANSWER: 630 is 7% of 9,000.

Once again, it can be seen that you multiply by 100 and using the same terms as before (**base** would equal the larger number and **amount** the smaller number), a simple formula can be devised:

$$\text{per cent} = \frac{100}{\text{base}} \times \text{amount } or \frac{\text{amount}}{\text{base}} \times 100$$

TIP BOX

In this case, **multiply** by 100 (it is always on the top line).

PROBLEMS

Work out the following:

Question 1   30% of 3,090

Question 2   84% of 42,825

Question 3   56.25% of 800

Question 4   60% of 80.6

Question 5   17.5% of 285.76

What percentage is:

Question 6   60 of 750 ?

Question 7   53,865 of 64,125 ?

Question 8   29.61 of 47 ?

Question 9   53.69 of 191.75 ?

Question 10   48 of 142 ?

Answers can be found on page 184

DRUG CALCULATIONS INVOLVING PERCENTAGES

The principles illustrated here can easily be applied to drug calculations. As before, it is unlikely that you will need to find the percentage of something, but these calculations are included here in order to gain an understanding of per cent and percentages, especially where drugs are concerned. Always, convert everything to the same units before doing the calculation.

WORKED EXAMPLE

What volume (in mL) is 60% of 1.25 litres?

Work in the same units – in this case, work in millilitres as these are the units required in the answer:

To convert to millilitres, multiply by 1,000 (see 'Chapter 4 Units and Equivalences' for a full explanation).

$$1.25 \text{ litres} = (1.25 \times 1,0000)\text{mL} = 1,250\text{mL}$$

Remember the number or quantity you want to find the percentage of is always equal to 100%.

$$1,250\text{mL} = 100\%$$

(You are converting the volume to a percentage.) Thus:

$$1\% = \frac{1,250}{100}$$

$$60\% = \frac{1,250}{100} \times 60 = 750\text{mL}$$

ANSWER: 60% of 1.25 litres is 750 mL.

Alternatively, you can use the formula:

$$\text{amount} = \frac{\text{base}}{100} \times \text{per cent}$$

Re-writing this as:

$$\frac{\text{what you've got}}{100} \times \text{percentage required}$$

where 'what you've got' = 1,250 mL and the percentage required = 60%.

Substitute the numbers into the formula:

$$\frac{1,250}{100} \times 60 = 750\,\text{mL}$$

ANSWER: 60% of 1.25 litres is 750 mL

Now consider the following example:

WORKED EXAMPLE

What percentage is 125 mg of 500 mg?

Everything is already in the same units, milligrams (mg), so there is no need for any conversions. As always, the quantity you want to find the percentage of is equal to 100%, i.e.

$$500\,\text{mg} = 100\%$$

(You are converting the amount to a percentage.) Thus:

$$1\,\text{mg} = \frac{100}{500}\%$$

$$125\,\text{mg} = \frac{100}{500} \times 125 = 25\%$$

ANSWER: 125 mg is 25% of 500 mg.

Alternatively, you can use the formula:

$$\text{per cent} = \frac{100}{\text{base}} \times \text{amount} \ \ or \ \ \frac{\text{amount}}{\text{base}} \times 100$$

where amount = 125 mg and base = 500 mg.

Substitute the numbers into the formula:

$$\frac{100}{500} \times 125 = 25\%$$

ANSWER: 125 mg is 25% of 500 mg.

HOW TO USE THE PERCENTAGE KEY ON YOUR CALCULATOR

Basic calculators are designed for everyday use and the percentage key [%] is designed as a shortcut so that calculation is not necessary. The percentage key [%] should be considered as a function and not as an operation such as add, subtract, multiply or divide.

Using the percentage key [%] automatically multiplies by 100. It is also important that the numbers and the percentage key [%] are pressed in the correct sequence; otherwise it is quite easy to get the wrong answer!

Let us go back to our original example: how much is 28% of 250?

You could easily find the answer by the long method, i.e.

$$\frac{250}{100} \times 28$$

Key in the sequence: [2][5][0] [÷] [1][0][0] [×] [2][8] [=], to give an answer of 70. This is exactly the calculation performed by the percentage key [%].

But when using the percentage key [%], you need to enter the following:

ENTER	[2][5][0]	DISPLAY = 250
ENTER	[×]	DISPLAY = 250
ENTER	[2][8]	DISPLAY = 28
ENTER	[%]	DISPLAY = 70 (answer)
ENTER	[=]	DISPLAY = 17500

Depending upon which calculator you have, pressing the [=] button may give the wrong answer!

What happens is, that by pressing the [=] button, you are multiplying 250 by 28% of 250 (i.e. by the answer):

250 × 28% of 250   or   250 × 70 = 17,500 (Giving a nonsensical answer!)

To make things easier, you can refer to the formulae derived from the worked examples. To find the amount a percentage is of a given quantity or number, we used the following formula:

$$\text{amount} = \frac{\text{base}}{100} \times \text{per cent}$$

The thing to remember is to **multiply**: [2][5][0] [×] [2][8] [%]

It also reminds us in which order to enter the numbers.

REMEMBER

Pressing the **per cent key [%] finishes** the current calculation. Thus when using the per cent key, **do not press the [=] button**.

Let us now look at the second example. What percentage is 630 of 9,000?

Once again, you can easily find the answer using the calculation:

$$\frac{630}{9,000} \times 100$$

Key in the sequence [6][3][0] [÷] [9][0][0][0] [×] [1][0][0] [=] to give an answer of 7%.

But when using the [%] button, you need to enter the following:

ENTER	[6][3][0]	DISPLAY = 630
ENTER	[÷]	DISPLAY = 630
ENTER	[9][0][0][0]	DISPLAY = 9000
ENTER	[%]	DISPLAY = 7% (answer)
ENTER	[=]	DISPLAY = 0.0007777

Once again, pressing the [=] button may give the wrong answer! What happens is that by pressing the [=] button, you are dividing by 9,000 again, i.e.:

$$\frac{630}{9,000 \times 9,000} \times 100$$

Once again, you can refer to the formulae derived from the worked examples. To find the percentage a number is of a given quantity or number, we used the following formula:

$$\text{per cent} = \frac{\text{amount}}{\text{base}} \times 100$$

The thing to remember is to **divide**: [6][3][0] [÷][9][0][0][0] [%].

Once again, it reminds us in which order to enter the numbers.
   Entering numbers in the wrong sequence gives us the wrong answer:

ENTER	[9][0][0][0]	DISPLAY = 9000
ENTER	[÷]	DISPLAY = 630
ENTER	[6][3][0]	DISPLAY = 630
ENTER	[%]	DISPLAY = 1428.5714
If you enter [=]:		
ENTER	[=]	DISPLAY = 2.2675736

To explain this, let us look at the long method of solving this problem:

$$9,000 = 100\%$$

Therefore:
$$1 = \frac{100}{9,000}\%$$

Thus:
$$630 = \frac{100}{9,000} \times 630\% \quad or \quad \frac{630}{9,000} \times 100\%$$

You can see that it is 630 **divided** by 9,000, and not the other way round.
   Therefore it is important to enter the numbers the right way round on your calculator.
   If you can't remember which way round to enter the numbers, an easy way to remember is: enter the **smaller** number (i.e. the **amount**) first.
   Also **remember**, pressing the **per cent key** [%] **finishes** the current calculation. Thus when using your calculator, **do not press the** [=] **button**.

To summarize, if you want to use the [%] button on your calculator, remember the following:

1 Enter the numbers in the right sequence.
  If you are finding the percentage of something, **multiply** the two numbers. (It doesn't matter in which order you enter the numbers.)
  If you are finding the percentage one number is of another, **divide** the **smaller** number (enter it first) by the **larger** number (enter it second). In this case, the sequence of numbers is important.
2 Always enter or press the [%] button **last**.
3 Do **not** enter or press the [=] button.
4 Refer to your calculator manual to see how your own calculator uses the [%] button.
5 Don't forget to clear your calculator (press the [CE] button), otherwise the numbers left in your calculator may be carried over to your next calculation.

Although using the [%] button is a quick way of finding percentages, you have to use it properly, therefore it may be best to ignore it; do the calculations the long way.

TIP BOX

Get to know how to use your calculator – read the manual! If you don't know how to use your calculator properly, then there is the potential for errors. You won't know if the answer you've got is correct or not.

At the end of this chapter, you should be familiar with the following:
- SI units
- Prefixes used in clinical medicine
- Equivalences
  - Equivalences of weight
  - Equivalences of volume
  - Equivalences of amount of substance
- Conversion from one unit to another
- Writing units

KEY POINTS

Equivalences of weight

UNIT	SYMBOL	EQUIVALENT	SYMBOL
1 kilogram	kg	1,000 grams	g
1 gram	g	1,000 milligrams	mg
1 milligram	mg	1,000 micrograms	mcg
1 microgram	mcg	1,000 nanograms	ng

Equivalences of volume

UNIT	SYMBOL	EQUIVALENT	SYMBOL
1 litre	L or l	1,000 millilitres	mL or ml

Equivalences of amount of substance

UNIT	SYMBOL	EQUIVALENT	SYMBOL
1 mole	mol	1,000 millimoles	mmol
1 millimole	mmol	1,000 micromoles	mcmol

- Milligrams, micrograms and nanograms should be written in full to avoid confusion.
- Avoid decimals: a decimal point written in the wrong place can mean 10-fold or even 100-fold errors.

Converting Units
- It is best to work with the smaller unit to avoid the use of decimals.
- When converting, the amount remains the same, only the unit changes.

> * Remember to look at the units carefully; converting from one unit to another may involve several steps.
> * To convert from a **larger** unit to the next **smaller** unit, **multiply** by 1,000.
> * To convert from a **smaller** unit to the next **larger** unit, **divide** by 1,000.

INTRODUCTION

Many different units are used in medicine, for example:

* drug strengths, e.g. digoxin injection 500 micrograms in 1 mL;
* dosages, e.g. dobutamine 3 mcg/kg/min;
* patient electrolyte levels, e.g. sodium 137 mmol/L.

It is important to have a basic knowledge of the units used in medicine and how they are derived.

It is particularly important to have an understanding of the units in which drugs can be prescribed, and how to convert from one unit to another – this last part is very important as it forms the basis of all drug calculations.

SI UNITS

SI stands for *Système Internationale (d'Unités)*, and is another name for the metric system of measurement. The aim of metrication is to make calculations easier than with the imperial system (ounces, pounds, stones, inches, pints, etc.). SI units are generally accepted in the United Kingdom and many other countries for use in medical practice and pharmacy. They were introduced in the NHS in 1975.

SI base units

The main units are those used to measure weight, volume and amount of substance:

* Weight: kilogram (kg)
* Volume: litre (l or L)
* Amount of substance: mole (mol)

SI prefixes

When an SI unit is inconveniently large or small, prefixes are used to denote multiples or sub-multiples. It is preferable to use multiples of a thousand. For example:

- gram
- milligram (one-thousandth, 1/1,000 of a gram)
- microgram (one-millionth, 1/1,000,000 of a gram)
- nanogram (one-thousand-millionth, 1/1,000,000,000 of a gram).

For example, one-millionth of a gram could be written as 0.000001 g or as 1 microgram. The second version is easier to read than the first and easier to work with once you understand how to use units and prefixes. It is also less likely to lead to errors, especially when administering drug doses.

PREFIXES USED IN CLINICAL MEDICINE

PREFIX	SYMBOL	DIVISION/MULTIPLE	FACTOR
Mega	M	× 1,000,000	10^6
Kilo	k	× 1,000	10^3
Deci	d	÷ 10	10^{-1}
Centi	c	÷ 100	10^{-2}
Milli	m	÷ 1,000	10^{-3}
Micro	mc (or μ)	÷ 1,000,000	10^{-6}
Nano	n	÷ 1,000,000,000	10^{-9}

The main prefixes you will come across on the ward are **mega-**, **milli-**, **micro-** and **nano-**. Thus, in practice, drug strengths and dosages can be expressed in various ways:

- Benzylpenicillin quantities are sometimes expressed in terms of mega-units (1 mega-unit means 1 million units of activity). Each vial contains benzylpenicillin 600 mg, which equals 1 mega-unit.
- Small volumes of liquids are often expressed in millilitres (mL) and are used to describe small dosages, e.g. lactulose, 10 mL to be given three times a day.
- Drug strengths are usually expressed in milligrams (mg), e.g. furosemide (frusemide) 40 mg tablets.
- When the amount of drug in a tablet or other formulation is very small, strengths are expressed in micrograms or even nanograms, e.g. digoxin 125 microgram tablets; alfacalcidol 250 nanogram capsules.

TIP BOX

In prescriptions the word 'micrograms' and 'nanograms' should be written in full. However, the abbreviation *mcg* (for micrograms) and *ng* (nanograms) are still sometimes used, so care must be taken when reading handwritten abbreviations. Confusion can occur, particularly between 'mg' and 'ng'. The old abbreviation of 'μg' should not be used as it may be confused with mg or ng.

EQUIVALENCES

The SI base units are too large for everyday clinical use, so they are subdivided into multiples of 1,000.

Equivalences of weight

UNIT	SYMBOL	EQUIVALENT	SYMBOL
1 kilogram	kg	1,000 grams	g
1 gram	g	1,000 milligrams	mg
1 milligram	mg	1,000 micrograms	mcg
1 microgram	mcg	1,000 nanograms	ng

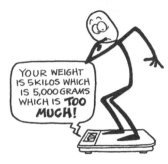

Equivalences of volume

UNIT	SYMBOL	EQUIVALENT	SYMBOL
1 litre	L or l*	1,000 millilitres	mL or ml

* See section on 'Guide to writing units' below.

Equivalences of amount of substance

UNIT	SYMBOL	EQUIVALENT	SYMBOL
1 mole	mol	1,000 millimoles	mmol
1 millimole	mmol	1,000 micromoles	mcmol

Moles and millimoles are the terms used by chemists when measuring quantities of certain substances or chemicals; they are more accurate than using grams. For a fuller explanation, see Chapter 7 on 'Moles and millimoles' (page 94).

Examples of eqivalent amounts include:

$$0.5\,kg = 500\,g$$
$$0.25\,g = 250\,mg$$
$$0.2\,mg = 200\,mcg$$
$$0.5\,L = 500\,mL$$
$$0.25\,mol = 250\,mmol$$

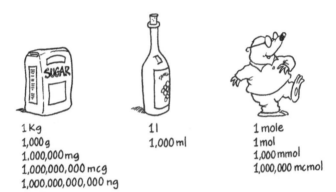

1 Kg	1 l	1 mole
1,000 g	1,000 ml	1 mol
1,000,000 mg		1,000 mmol
1,000,000,000 mcg		1,000,000 mcmol
1,000,000,000,000 ng		

CONVERSION FROM ONE UNIT TO ANOTHER

In drug calculations, it is best to work in whole numbers, i.e. 125 micrograms rather than 0.125 mg, as fewer mistakes are then made. Avoid using decimals, as the decimal point can be written in the wrong place during calculations. A decimal point in the wrong place can mean 10-fold or even 100-fold errors.

It is always best to work with the smaller unit in order to avoid decimals and decimal points, so you need to be able to convert easily from one unit to another. In general:

• To convert from a **larger** unit to a **smaller** unit, **multiply** by multiples of 1,000.
• To convert from a **smaller** unit to a **larger** unit, **divide** by multiples of 1,000.

For each multiplication or division by 1,000, the decimal point moves three places, either to the right or left depending upon whether you are converting from a larger unit to a smaller unit or vice versa.

There are two methods for converting units: moving the decimal point or by using boxes which is an easy way to multiply or divide by a thousand (see the worked examples below).

When you have to convert from a very large unit to a much smaller unit (or vice versa), you may find it easier to do the conversion in several steps.

For example, to convert 0.005 kg to milligrams, first convert to grams:

$$0.005\,kg = (0.005 \times 1,000)g = 5\,g$$

Next, convert grams to milligrams:

$$5\,g = (5 \times 1,000)\,mg = 5,000\,mg$$

REMEMBER

When you do conversions like this, the amount remains the same: it is only the units that change. Obviously, it appears more when expressed as a smaller unit, but the **amount remains the same**. (200 pence is the same as £2, although it may look more.)

WORKED EXAMPLE
Convert 0.5 g to milligrams.

METHOD ONE: MOVING THE DECIMAL POINT
You are going from a larger unit to a smaller unit, so you have to *multiply* by 1,000, i.e.

$$0.5 \times 1,000 = 500 \text{ milligrams}$$

The **decimal point** moves **three** places to the **right**:

$$0 \overset{\frown}{\cdot} 5\ 0\ 0 = 500$$

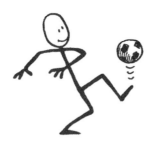

METHOD TWO: USING BOXES
Place the higher unit in the **left-hand** box and the smaller unit in the **right-hand** box:

g			mg

Next place an arrow between the units pointing from the unit you are converting from towards the unit you are going to. In this example, we are converting from grams (g) to milligrams (mg), so the arrow will point from **left** to **right**:

g	→	mg

Next enter the numbers into the boxes, starting from the column of the unit you are converting from, i.e. in this example, it will be the **left-hand** side. Enter the numbers 0 and 5 (0.5 kg):

g	→	mg
0	5	

Place zeros in any empty boxes

g	→	mg
0	5	0	0

Now we have to decide where to place the decimal point. Remember, when converting units you either multiply or divide by 1,000 (or multiples thereof). The decimal point moves **three** places to the **left** or the **right**. The arrow indicates which way the decimal point moves. In this case, it is pointing to the **right**, so starting at the right of the original place of the decimal point, add the numbers 1, 2 and 3 in the boxes:

g	→	mg
0	5	0	0
	1	2	3

The decimal point is then placed to the right of the 3, giving an answer of 500. Add the new unit, mg, to get a final answer:

g	→	mg
0	5	0	0	.
	1	2	3	

So the answer is 500 milligrams.

WORKED EXAMPLE

Convert 2,000 g to kilograms.

METHOD ONE: MOVING THE DECIMAL POINT

You are going from a smaller unit to a larger unit, so you have to *divide* by 1,000, i.e.

$$2,000\,g = \left(\frac{2,000}{1,000} \right) kg = 2\,kg$$

The **decimal point** moves **three** places to the **left**:

$$2\,0\,0\,0. = 2\,kg$$

METHOD TWO: USING BOXES

Place the higher unit in the **left-hand** box and the smaller unit in the **right-hand** box:

kg			g

Next place an arrow between the units pointing from the unit you are converting from towards the unit you are going to. In this example, we are converting from grams (g) to kilograms (kg), so the arrow will point from **right** to **left**:

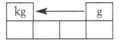

Next enter the numbers into the boxes as seen, starting from the unit you are converting from, i.e. in this example from the **right-hand** side:

kg ◄—		g
◄—	0	0

So, the numbers are written 0, 0, 0 and 2 to give 2,000 g:

kg ◄—			g
2	0	0	0

Now we have to decide where to place the decimal point. We are converting from grams (g) to kilograms (kg), so the arrow is pointing from **right** to **left**. Enter the numbers 1, 2 and 3 according to the direction of the arrow:

kg	←		g
2	0	0	0
	3	2	1

Place the decimal point after the figure 3; in this case it goes between the 2 and the first 0:

kg	←		g
2	0	0	0
.	3	2	1

Add the new units (kg), giving an answer of 2 kilograms

WORKED EXAMPLE

Convert 150 nanograms to micrograms.

METHOD ONE: MOVING THE DECIMAL POINT

You are going from a smaller unit to a larger unit, so you have to *divide* by 1,000, i.e.

$$\frac{150}{1,000} \text{ nanograms} = 0.150 \text{ micrograms}$$

The **decimal point** moves **three** places to the **left**:

$$0 \overset{\frown}{.} 1\ 5\ 0 = 0.150$$

METHOD TWO: USING BOXES

Place the higher unit in the **left-hand** box and the smaller unit in the **right-hand** box:

mcg			ng

Next, add an arrow pointing in the direction of the conversion:

mcg	←		ng

Next enter the numbers into the boxes, starting from the unit you are converting from, i.e. in this example from the **right-hand** side: the numbers are 0, 5 and 1 to give 150 nanograms:

mcg	←		ng
	1	5	0

Place a zero in any empty boxes:

mcg			ng
0	1	5	0

Now we have to decide where to place the decimal point. We are converting from nanograms (ng) to micrograms (mcg), so the arrow is pointing from **right** to **left**. Enter the numbers 1, 2 and 3 according to the direction of the arrow:

mcg			ng
0	1	5	0
	3	*2*	*1*

Place the decimal point after the figure 3; in this case it goes between the 0 and the 1:

mcg			ng
0	1	5	0
.	*3*	*2*	*1*

Add the new units (mcg), giving an answer of 0.150 micrograms.

GUIDE TO WRITING UNITS

The *British National Formulary* makes the following recommendations:

- The unnecessary use of decimal points should be avoided, e.g. 3 mg, **not** 3.0 mg.
- Quantities of 1 gram or more should be expressed as 1.5 g, etc.
- Quantities less than 1 gram should be written in milligrams, e.g. 500 mg, **not** 0.5 g.
- Quantities less than 1 mg should be written in micrograms, e.g. 100 micrograms, **not** 0.1 mg.
- When decimals are unavoidable, a zero should be written in front of the decimal point where there is no other figure, e.g. 0.5 mL **not** .5 mL. However, the use of a decimal point is acceptable to express a range, e.g. 0.5–1 g.
- Micrograms and nanograms should **not** be abbreviated. Similarly, 'units' should **not** be abbreviated.
- A capital L is used for litre, to avoid confusion (a small letter l could be mistaken for a figure 1 (one), especially when typed or printed).
- Cubic centimetre, or cm^3, is **not** used in medicine or pharmacy; use millilitre (mL or ml) instead.

The following two case reports illustrate how bad writing can lead to problems.

CONFUSING MICROGRAMS AND MILLIGRAMS

Case report

On admission to hospital, a patient taking thyroxine replacement therapy presented her general practitioner's referral letter which stated that her maintenance dose was 0.025 mg once daily. The clerking house officer incorrectly converted this dose and prescribed 250 micrograms rather than the 25 micrograms required. A dose was administered before the error was detected by the ward pharmacist the next morning.

Taken from: *Pharmacy in Practice 1994; **4**: 124.*

This example highlights several errors:
- The wrong units were originally used – milligrams instead of micrograms.
- A number containing a decimal points was used.
- Conversion from one unit to another was carried out incorrectly.

THIS UNIT ABBREVIATION IS DANGEROUS

Case report

Patient received 50 units of insulin instead of the prescribed stat dose of 5 units. A junior doctor requiring a patient to be given a stat dose of 5 units Actrapid insulin wrote the prescription appropriately but chose to incorporate the abbreviation ☉ for 'units', which is occasionally seen used on written requests for units of blood. Thus the prescription read: 'Actrapid insulin 5☉ stat'.

The administering nurse misread the abbreviation and interpreted the prescription as 50 units of insulin. This was administered to the patient, who of course became profoundly hypoglycaemic and required urgent medical intervention.

Comment

The use of the symbol ☉ to indicate units of blood is an old-fashioned practice which is now in decline. This case serves to illustrate the catastrophic effect that the inappropriate use of this abbreviation can have – it led to misinterpretation by the nursing staff and resulted in harm to the patient.

Taken from: *Pharmacy in Practice 1995; **5**: 131.*

This example illustrates that abbreviations should not be used. As recommended, the word 'units' should **not** be abbreviated.

PROBLEMS

Question 1	Convert 0.0125 kilograms to grams.
Question 2	Convert 250 nanograms to micrograms.
Question 3	Convert 3.2 litres to millilitres.
Question 4	Convert 0.0273 moles to millimoles.
Question 5	Convert 3,750 grams to kilograms.
Question 6	Convert 0.05 grams to micrograms.
Question 7	Convert 25,000 milligrams to kilograms.
Question 8	Convert 4.5×10^{-6} grams to nanograms.
Question 9	You have an ampoule of digoxin 0.25 mg/mL.
	Calculate the amount of digoxin in micrograms in a 2 mL ampoule.
Question 10	You have an ampoule of fentanyl 0.05 mg/mL.
	Calculate the amount of fentanyl in micrograms in a 2 mL ampoule.

Answers can be found on page 184.

OBJECTIVES

At the end of this chapter, you should be familiar with the following:

- Percentage concentration
  - Calculating the total amount of drug in a solution
- mg/ml concentration
  - Converting percentage to a mg/ml concentration
- 'I in ...' concentrations or ratio strengths
- Parts per million (ppm)
- Drug concentrations expressed in units: heparin and insulin

---

KEY POINTS

Percentage Concentration

% w/v = number of grams in 100 mL

(A solid is dissolved in a liquid, thus 5% w/v means 5 g in 100 mL.)

% w/w = number of grams in 100 g

(A solid mixed with another solid, thus 5% w/w means 5 g in 100 g.)

%v/v = number of mL in 100 mL

(A liquid is mixed or diluted with another liquid, thus 5% v/v means 5 mL in 100 mL.)

- Most common percentage strength encountered is % w/v.
- There will always be the same amount of drug present in 100 mL irrespective of the total volume. Thus in a 5% w/v solution, there is 5 g dissolved in each 100 mL of fluid and this will remain the same if it is a 500 mL bag or a 1 litre bag.
- To find the total amount of drug present, the total volume must be taken into account – in 500 mL of a 5% w/v solution there is a total of 25 g present.

mg/mL Concentrations

- Defined as the number of milligrams of drug per millilitre of liquid.
- Oral liquids – usually expressed as the number of mg in a standard 5 mL spoonful, e.g. erythromycin 250 mg in 5 mL.
- Injections are usually expressed as the number of mg per volume of the ampoule (1 mL, 2 mL, 5 mL, 10 mL or 20 mL), e.g. gentamicin 80 mg in 2 mL.

Strengths can also be expressed in mcg/mL.

Converting percentage concentrations to mg/mL concentrations

- Multiply the percentage by 10, e.g. lidocaine (lignocaine) 0.2% = 2 mg/mL.

Converting mg/mL concentratios to percentage concentrations
- Divide the mg/mL strength by 10, e.g. lidocaine (lignocaine) 2 mg/mL = 2%.

'I in ...' Concentrations or Ratio Strengths
- Defined as: **one** gram in however many millilitres.

For example:

I in 1,000 means 1 g in 1,000 mL

I in 10,000 means 1 g in 10,000 mL

Parts per Million (ppm)
- Similar to ratio strengths, but used to describe very dilute concentrations.
- Most common ppm concentration encountered is that of a solid dissolved in a liquid, but can also apply to two solids or liquids mixed together.
- Defined as: **one** gram in 1,000,000 mL *or* **one** milligram in 1 litre.

Units – Heparin and Insulin
- The purity of drugs such as insulin and heparin from animal or biosynthetic sources varies.
- Therefore these drugs are expressed in terms of **units** as a standard measurement rather than weight.

INTRODUCTION

There are various ways of expressing how much actual drug is present in a medicine. These medicines are usually liquids that are for oral or parenteral administration, but also include those for topical use.

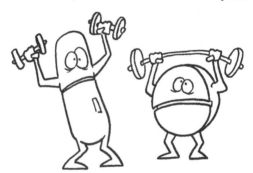

The aim of this chapter is to explain the various ways in which drug strengths can be stated.

PERCENTAGE CONCENTRATION

Following on from the last chapter, one method of describing concentration is to use the percentage as a unit. Percentage concentration can be defined as the amount of drug in 100 parts of the product.

The most common method you will come across is the percentage concentration w/v (weight in volume). This is used when a solid is dissolved in a liquid and means the number of grams dissolved in 100 mL:

% w/v = number of grams in 100 mL

(Thus 5% w/v means 5 g in 100 mL.)

Another type of concentration you might come across is the percentage concentration w/w (weight in weight). This is used when a solid is mixed with another solid, e.g. in creams and ointments, and means the number of grams in 100 g:

% w/w = number of grams in 100 g

(Thus 5% w/w means 5 g in 100 g.)

Another is the percentage concentration v/v (volume in volume). This is used when a liquid is mixed or diluted with another liquid, and means the number of millilitres (mL) in 100 mL:

% v/v = number of mL in 100 mL

(Thus 5% v/v means 5 mL in 100 mL.)

The most common percentage concentration you will encounter is the percentage w/v or 'weight in volume' and therefore this will be the one considered here.

In our earlier example of 5% w/v, there are 5 g in 100 mL irrespective of the size of the container. For example, glucose 5% infusion means that there are 5 g of glucose dissolved in each 100 mL of fluid and this will remain the same if it is a 500 mL bag or a 1 litre bag.

To find the total amount of drug present in a bottle or infusion bag, you must take into account the size or volume of the bottle or infusion bag.

WORKED EXAMPLE

TO CALCULATE THE TOTAL AMOUNT OF DRUG IN A SOLUTION
How much sodium bicarbonate is there in a 200 mL infusion sodium bicarbonate 8.4% w/v?

STEP ONE
Convert the percentage to the number of grams in 100 mL, i.e.

8.4% w/v = 8.4 g in 100 mL

(You are converting the percentage to a specific quantity.)

STEP TWO

Calculate how many grams there are in 1 mL, i.e. divide by 100:

$$\frac{8.4\,\text{g}}{100} \text{ in 1 mL (using the 'ONE unit' rule)}$$

STEP THREE

However, you have a 200 mL infusion. So to find out the total amount present, multiply how much is in 1 mL by the volume you've got (200 mL):

$$\frac{8.4}{100} \times 200 = 16.8\,\text{g in 200 mL}$$

ANSWER: There are 16.8 g of sodium bicarbonate in 200 mL of sodium bicarbonate 8.4% w/v infusion.

A simple formula can be devised based upon the formula seen earlier:

$$\text{amount} = \frac{\text{base}}{100} \times \text{per cent}$$

This can be re-written as:

$$\text{total amount (g)} = \frac{\text{percentage}}{100} \times \text{total volume (mL)}$$

Therefore in this example:

$$\text{Percentage} = 8.4$$
$$\text{Total volume (mL)} = 200$$

Substituting the numbers into the formula:

$$\text{Total amount (g)} = \frac{8.4}{100} \times 200 = 16.8\,\text{g}$$

ANSWER: There are 16.8 g of sodium bicarbonate in 200 mL of sodium bicarbonate 8.4% w/v infusion.

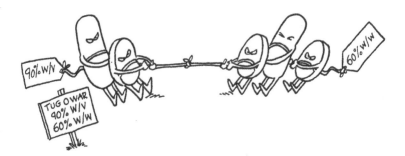

PROBLEMS

Calculate how many grams there are in the following:

Question 1   How many grams of sodium chloride are there in a litre infusion of sodium chloride 0.9%?

Question 2   How many grams of potassium, sodium and glucose are there in a litre infusion of potassium 0.3%, sodium chloride 0.18% and glucose 4%?

Question 3   How many grams of sodium chloride are there in a 500 mL infusion of sodium chloride 0.45%?

Question 4   You need to give calcium gluconate 2 g as a slow intravenous injection.

You have 10 mL ampoules of calcium gluconate 10%.

How much do you need to draw up?

Answers can be found on page 187.

mg/mL CONCENTRATIONS

Another way of expressing the amount or concentration of drug in a solution, usually for oral or parenteral administration, is in mg/mL, i.e. number of milligrams of drug per mL of liquid. This is the most common way of expressing the amount of drug in a solution.

For oral liquids, it is usually expressed as the number of milligrams in a standard 5 mL spoonful, e.g. amoxicillin (amoxycillin) 250 mg in 5 mL.

For oral doses that are less than 5 mL an oral syringe would be used (see the section 'Administration of medicines' in Chapter 9 'Action and administration of medicines', page xx).

For injections, it is usually expressed as the number of milligrams per volume of the ampoule (1 mL, 2 mL, 5 mL, 10 mL and 20 mL), e.g. gentamicin 80 mg in 2 mL. However, injections may still be expressed as the number of milligrams per mL, e.g. furosemide (frusemide) 10 mg/mL, 2 mL – particularly in old reference sources.

Note: Strengths can also be expressed in mcg/mL, e.g. hyoscine injection 600 mcg/1 mL. Only mg/mL will be considered here, but the principles learnt here can be applied to other concentrations or strengths, e.g. mcg/mL. Sometimes it may be useful to convert percentage concentrations to mg/mL concentrations. For example:

lidocaine 0.2%	= 0.2 g per 100 mL
(lignocaine)	= 200 mg per 100 mL
	= 2 mg per mL (2 mg/mL)
sodium chloride 0.9%	= 0.9 g per 100 mL
	= 900 mg per 100 mL
	= 9 mg per mL (9 mg/mL)
glucose 5%	= 5 g per 100 mL
	= 5,000 mg per 100 mL
	= 50 mg per mL (50 mg/mL)

This will give the strength of the solution irrespective of the size of the bottle, infusion bag, etc.

If you know the percentage concentration, an easy way of finding the strength in mg/mL is by simply multiplying the percentage by 10.

This can be explained using lidocaine (lignocaine) 0.2% as an example: You have lidocaine (lignocaine) 0.2% – this is equal to 0.2 g in 100 mL. Divide by 100 to find out how much is in 1 mL. Thus:

$$\frac{0.2}{100} \text{ g/mL}$$

Multiply by 1,000 to convert grams to milligrams. Thus:

$$\frac{0.2}{100} \times 1,000 \text{ mg/mL}$$

Simplify the above calculation to give:

$$0.2 \times 10 = 2 \text{ mg/mL}$$

Therefore you simply multiply the percentage by 10.

With the other examples above:

sodium chloride 0.9%	$0.9 \times 10 = 9 \text{ mg/mL}$
glucose 5%	$5 \times 10 = 50 \text{ mg/mL}$

Conversely, to convert a mg/mL concentration to a percentage, you simply divide by 10.

Once again, if we use our original lidocaine (lignocaine) as an example: You have lidocaine (lignocaine) 2 mg/mL.

Percentage means 'per 100 mL', so multiply by 100, i.e.

$$2 \text{ mg/mL} \times 100 = 200 \text{ mg/100 mL} (2 \times 100)$$

Remember, percentage (w/v) means 'the number of grams per 100 mL', so you will have to convert milligrams to grams by dividing by 1,000, i.e.

$$\frac{2 \times 100}{1,000} = \frac{2}{10} = 0.2\%$$

Therefore to change a strength in mg/mL to a percentage strength you simply divide the mg/mL concentration by 10.

With our other examples:

sodium chloride 9 mg/mL   9 ÷ 10 = 0.9%
glucose 50 mg/mL   50 ÷ 10 = 5%

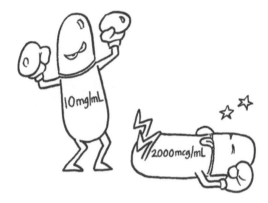

PROBLEMS

Calculate the strengths (mg/mL) for the following:

Question 5   Sodium chloride infusion 0.45%

Question 6   Metronidazole infusion 0.5%

Question 7   Potassium chloride 0.2%, sodium chloride 0.18% and glucose 4%

Convert the following mg/mL strengths to percentage strengths:

Question 8   Bupivacaine 2.5 mg/mL

Question 9   Glucose 500 mg/mL

Question 10   Isosorbide dinitrate 500 micrograms/mL

Answers can be found on page 187.

'I IN ...' CONCENTRATIONS OR RATIO STRENGTHS

This style of expressing concentration is used only occasionally, and is written as 'I in ...', e.g. 1 in 10,000, and is sometimes known as a ratio strength. It usually refers to a solid dissolved in a liquid and, by agreed convention, the weight is expressed in grams and the volume in millilitres.

So, it means **one** gram in however many mL. For example:

'1 in 1,000' means 1 g in 1,000 mL
'1 in 10,000' means 1 g in 10,000 mL

Therefore it can be seen that 1 in 10,000 is weaker than 1 in 1,000. So, the higher the 'number', the weaker the solution.

The drug most commonly expressed this way is adrenaline/epinephrine:

Adrenaline/epinephrine 1 in 1,000 which is equal to 1 *mg* in 1 mL
Adrenaline/epinephrine 1 in 10,000 which is equal to 1 *mg* in 10 mL

An easy way to remember the above is to cancel out the three zeros that appear after the comma, i.e.

Adrenaline/epinephrine 1 in 1,000 –
cancel out the three zeros after the comma: 1,∅∅∅ to give:
1 in 1 which can be written as: 1 mg in 1 mL

Similarly, for adrenaline/epinephrine 1 in 10,000 – cancel out the three zeros after the comma: 10,∅∅∅ to give: 1 in 10, which can be written as 1 mg in 10 mL.

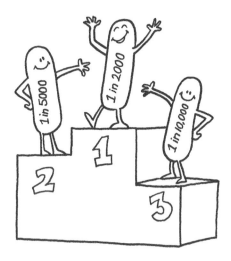

PARTS PER MILLION (ppm)

This is a way of expressing very dilute concentrations. Just as per cent means parts of a hundred, so parts per million or ppm means parts of a million. It usually refers to a solid dissolved in a liquid but, as with percentage concentrations, it can also be used for two solids or two liquids mixed together.

Once again, by agreed convention:

I ppm means I g in 1,000,000 mL or I mg in I litre (1,000 mL)

In terms of percentage, 1 ppm equals 0.0001%.
Other equivalents include:

One part per million is one second in 12 days of your life!

One part per million is one penny out of £10,000!

For example, solutions produced by disinfectant chlorine-releasing agents (e.g. Haz-Tabs®) are measured in terms of parts per million, such as 1,000 ppm available chlorine.

PROBLEMS

Question 11   Adrenaline/epinephrine is sometimes combined with lidocaine (lignocaine) when used as a local anaesthetic, usually at a 1 in 200,000 strength. How much adrenaline/epinephrine is there in a 20 mL vial?

Question 12   It is recommended that children should have fluoride supplements for their teeth if the fluoride content of drinking water is 0.7 ppm or less. Express this concentration in micrograms per litre.

Answers can be found on page 188.

DRUGS EXPRESSED IN UNITS

Doses of drugs that are derived from large biological molecules are expressed in 'units' rather than weights. Such large molecules are difficult to purify and so, rather than use a weight, it is more accurate to use the biological activity of the drug, which is expressed in units. Examples of such drugs are heparin and insulin.

The calculation of doses and their translation into suitable dosage forms are similar to the calculations elsewhere in this chapter.

Heparin

Unfractionated heparin (UFH) is given subcutaneously or by continuous intravenous infusion. Infusions are usually given over 24 hours and the dose is adjusted according to laboratory results. However, low molecular weight heparins (LMWHs) differ from unfractionated heparin (UFH) in molecular size and weight, method of preparation and anticoagulant properties. The anticoagulant response to LMWH is highly correlated with body weight, allowing administration of a fixed dose, usually expressed in terms of a patient's body weight.

Confusion can occur between units and volume: the following case report illustrates the point that particular care must be taken when prescribing and administering LMWHs.

BEWARE DOSING ERRORS WITH LOW MOLECULAR WEIGHT HEPARIN

Case report

A retired teacher was admitted to hospital with acute shortage of breath and was diagnosed as having a pulmonary embolus. She was prescribed subcutaneous tinzaparin, in a dose of 0.45 mL from a 20,000 unit per mL pre-filled 0.5 mL syringe. Owing to confusion over the intended dose, two 0.5 mL prefilled syringes or 20,000 units of tinzaparin were administered in error by the ward nursing staff on four consecutive days. As a result of this cumulative administration error the patient died from a brain haemorrhage which, in the opinion of the pathologist, was due to the overdose of tinzaparin.

It was the prescriber's intention that the patient should receive 9,000 units of tinzaparin each day, but this information was not written on the prescription. The ward sister told a coroner's court hearing that the prescription was ambiguous. The dose was written as 0.45 mL and then 20,000 units, with the rest illegible. Owing to this confusion the patient received an overdose and died.

Taken from: *Pharmacy in Practice 2000; **10**: 260.*

Insulin

Injection devices ('pens'), which hold the insulin in a cartridge and deliver the required dose, are convenient to use. However, the conventional syringe and needle are still the method of insulin administration preferred by many and are also required for insulin not available in cartridge form.

There are no calculations involved in the administration of insulin. Insulin comes in cartridges or vials containing 100 units/mL, and the doses prescribed are written in units.

Therefore, all you have to do is to dial or draw up the required dose using a pen device or an insulin syringe.

Insulin syringes are calibrated as 100 units in 1 mL and are available as 1 mL and 0.5 mL syringes.

So if the dose is 30 units, you simply draw up to the 30 unit mark on the syringe.

PART II: Performing calculations

6 DOSAGE CALCULATIONS

OBJECTIVES

At the end of this chapter, you should be familiar with the following:

- Calculating the number of tablets or capsules required
- Dosages based on patient parameters
- Ways of expressing doses
- Calculating dosages
- Displacement values or volumes
  What is displacement?
  Is displacement important in medicine?

KEY POINTS

Calculating the Number of Tablets or Capsules Required

$$\text{number required} = \frac{\text{amount prescribed}}{\text{amount in each tablet or capsule}}$$

Dosages Based on Patient Parameters

- Weight (dose/kg): dose × body weight (kg)
- Surface area (dose/m^2): dose × body surface area (m^2)

Ways of Expressing Doses

A dose can be described as a:

- single dose – sometimes referred to as a 'stat' dose meaning 'at once' from the Latin *statum*
- daily dose: e.g. atorvastatin 10 mg once daily
  weekly dose: e.g. methotrexate, when used in rheumatoid arthritis
- divided or total daily dose: e.g. 12.5–25 mg/kg twice daily (total daily dose may alternatively be given in three or four divided doses)

Calculating Doses

$$\frac{\text{amount you want}}{\text{amount you've got}} \times \text{volume it's in}$$

- Take care when reading doses, either prescribed or found in the literature.
- Total daily dose (TDD) is the total dose and needs to be divided by the number of doses per day to give a single dose.
- To be sure that your answer is correct, it is best to calculate from first principles (for example, using the 'ONE unit' rule).
- If using a formula, make sure that the figures are entered correctly.
- Ensure that everything is in the same units.

• Ask yourself: does my answer seem reasonable?
• Always re-check your answer – if in any doubt, **stop** and get help.

Displacement Values or Volumes

• Dry powder injections need to be reconstituted with a diluent before they are used. Sometimes the final volume of the injection will be greater than the volume of liquid that was added to the powder. This volume difference is called the injection's displacement value.

Volume to be added = diluent volume – displacement volume

INTRODUCTION

Dosage calculations are the basic everyday type of calculations you will be doing on the ward. They include calculating number of tablets or capsules required, divided doses, simple drug dosages and dosages based on patient parameters, e.g. weight and body surface area.

It is important that you are able to do these calculations confidently, as mistakes may result in the patient receiving the wrong dose which may lead to serious consequences for the patient.

After completing this chapter, should you not only be able to do the calculations, but also be able to decide whether your answer is reasonable or not.

CALCULATING THE NUMBER OF TABLETS OR CAPSULES REQUIRED

On the drug round, you will usually have available the strength of the tablets or capsules for the dose prescribed on a patient's drug chart, e.g. dose prescribed is furosemide (frusemide) 40 mg; tablets available are furosemide (frusemide) 40 mg. However, there may be instances when the strength of the tablets or capsules available do not match the dose prescribed. Then you will have to calculate how many tablets or capsules to give the patient.

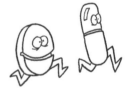

WORKED EXAMPLES

A patient is prescribed 75 mcg of levothyroxine sodium (thyroxine sodium) but the strength of the tablets available is 25 mcg. How many tablets are required?

This is a very simple calculation. The answer involves finding how many 25s there are in 75 or in other words 75 divided by 25:

$$\frac{75}{25} = \frac{3}{1} = 3 \text{ tablets}$$

In most cases, it is a simple sum you can do in your head, but even so, it is a drug calculation – so care must always be taken.

A patient is prescribed 2 g of flucloxacillin to be given orally but it is available in 500 mg capsules. How many capsules should you give?

Once again it is a simple calculation but it is slightly more complicated than our earlier example as the dose prescribed and the available medication are in different units.

The first step is to convert everything to the same units. We could either convert the 500 mg into grams, or we could convert the 2 g into milligrams.

In this case it is preferable to convert the grams to milligrams as this avoids decimal points. Remember it is best not to work with decimal points – a decimal point in the wrong place can mean a 10-fold or even a 100-fold error.

To convert grams to milligrams, multiply by 1,000:

$$2\,g = (2 \times 1,000)\,mg = 2,000\,mg$$

The calculation is now similar to our earlier example. The answer involves finding how many 500s are in 2,000 or in other words 2,000 divided by 500:

$$\frac{2,000}{500} = \frac{4}{1} = 4 \text{ capsules}$$

Once again, it is a simple sum you can do in your head, but it is a drug calculation, so care must always be taken.

A formula can be derived:

$$\text{number required} = \frac{\text{amount prescribed}}{\text{amount in each tablet or capsule}}$$

For dosage calculations involving liquids and injections, see the section 'Calculating drug dosages' on page 87.

PROBLEMS

Question 1   500 mg is prescribed and the tablets are 250 mg each. How many tablets will you give?

Question 2   Alfacalcidol 1 microgram is prescribed. If you only have 250 nanogram capsules, how many would you give?

Answers can be found on page 188.

DOSAGES BASED ON PATIENT PARAMETERS

Sometimes, the dose required is calculated on a body weight basis (mg/kg) or in terms of a patient's surface area (mg/m²). Using body surface area (BSA) estimates is more accurate than using body weight, since many physical phenomena are more closely related to BSA. This particularly applies to cytotoxics and other drugs that require an accurate individual dose. To find the BSA for a patient, you will need to know that patient's height and weight. Then the BSA can be calculated, using a formula or nomograms (see Appendix 1, page 217).

WORKED EXAMPLES

WEIGHT

The dose required is 3 mg/kg and the patient weighs 68 kg.

This means that for every kilogram (kg) of a patient's weight, you will need 3 mg of drug.

In this example, the patient weighs 68 kg.

Therefore this patient will need 68 lots of 3 mg of drug, i.e. you simply multiply the dose by the patient's weight:

$$3 \times 68 = 204 \, \text{mg}$$

Thus the patient will need a total dose of 204 mg.

This can be summarized as:

total dose required = dose per kg × patient's weight

SURFACE AREA

Doses are calculated in the same way, substituting surface area for weight.

For example: the dose required is 500 mg/m^2 and the patient's body surface area is 1.89 m^2.

For every square metre (m^2) of a patient's surface area, you will need 500 mg of drug.

In this example, the patient's body surface area is 1.89 m^2.

Therefore this patient will need 1.89 lots of 500 mg of drug, i.e. you simply multiply the dose by the patient's body surface area (obtained from a formula or nomograms – see Appendix 1).

$$500 \times 1.89 = 945 \, \text{mg}$$

Thus the patent will need a total dose of 945 mg.

This can be summarized as:

total dose required = dose per m^2 × body surface area

When using this method of calculation, the actual body weight should be used. However, in the case of obese children, the child may receive an artificially high dose. The reason for this is that fat tissue plays virtually no part in metabolism, and the dose must be estimated on lean or ideal body weight.

As a rule of thumb, doses should be reduced by approximately 25% for obese children.

PROBLEMS

Work out the following dosages:

Question 3   Dose = 1.5 mg/kg, patient's weight = 73 kg

Question 4   Dose = 60 mg/kg, patient's weight = 12 kg

Question 5   Dose = 50 mg/m^2, patient's surface area = 1.94 m^2

Question 6   Dose = 120 mg/m^2, patient's surface area = 1.55 m^2

Question 7   Dose = 400 mcg/kg, patient's weight = 54 kg

          i) What is the total dose in micrograms?

          ii) What is the total dose in mg?

Question 8   Dose = 5 mcg/kg/min, patient's weight = 65 kg

          What is the dose in mcg/min?

          (You will meet this type of calculation with IV infusions – see page 117.)

The following table will be needed to answer questions 9 and 10.

LMWH	STRENGTH	PREPARATIONS AVAILABLE
Enoxaparin (*Clexane*®)	100 mg/mL (10,000 units/mL)	0.2 mL syringe (2,000 units, 20 mg) 0.4 mL syringe (4,000 units, 40 mg) 0.6 mL syringe (6,000 units, 60 mg) 0.8 mL syringe (8,000 units, 80 mg) 1 mL syringe (10,000 units, 100 mg)
Tinzaparin (*Innohep*®)	20,000 units/mL	0.5 mL syringe (10,000 units) 0.7 mL syringe (14,000 units) 0.9 mL syringe (18,000 units) 2 mL vial (40,000 units)

Question 9   A patient has a deep vein thrombosis (DVT) and needs to be given tinzaparin at a dose of 175 units/kg. The patient weighs 68 kg. What dose do they need, which syringe do you use and volume you give?

Question 10 A patient has a DVT and has been prescribed enoxaparin 1.5 mg/kg. The patient weighs 59 kg. What dose do they need, which syringe do you use and volume you give?

Question 11   Using the Mosteller BSA formula (see Appendix 1):

$$\text{BSA m}^2 = \sqrt{\frac{\text{height (cm)} \times \text{weight (kg)}}{3,600}}$$

find out the body surface area for a child weighing 20 kg with a height of 108 cm.

Question 12   Using the Mosteller BSA formula (see Appendix 1):

$$\text{BSA m}^2 = \sqrt{\frac{\text{height (cm)} \times \text{weight (kg)}}{3,600}}$$

Find out the body surface area for a patient weighing 96 kg and with a height of 180 m.

Answers can be found on page 188.

WAYS OF EXPRESSING DOSES

A dose is the quantity or amount of a drug taken by, or administered to, a patient to achieve a therapeutic outcome.

A dose can be described as a **single** dose, a **daily** dose, a **daily divided** dose, a **weekly** dose or a **total** dose, etc., as described in the examples below:

- Single dose: for example, pre-medication drugs – this is sometimes referred to as a 'stat' dose, meaning 'at once' from the Latin *statum*.
- Daily dose: for example, the BNF recommended dose of atorvastatin is 10 mg once daily.
- Weekly dose: for example, methotrexate, when used in rheumatoid arthritis.
- Divided or total daily dose: for example, the *BNF for Children* recommends for cefradine (cephradine):

By mouth

Child 1 month–12 years

12.5–25 mg/kg **twice daily** (**total daily dose** may alternatively be given in three or four divided doses)

As stated above, the dose of a drug can be given as a total daily dose (TDD), which has to be given in divided doses (usually three or four times a day). This is particularly associated with paediatric doses.

It is important that you can tell the difference between the TDD and individual doses. If not interpreted properly, then the patient is at risk of receiving the TDD as an individual dose, thus receiving three or four times the normal dose (with potentially disastrous results).

Consider the above example for a 6-year-old (weight = 20.5 kg).

If giving a dose of cefradine (cephradine) 12.5 mg/kg, then the dose is 12.5 × 20.5 = 256mg (256 mg 'rounded up'). Consider the above example for a 6 year old weight = 20.5kg)

If giving a dose of cefradine (cephradine) 12.5 mg/kg, then the dose is $12.5 \times 20.5 = (256.25$ mg 'rounded down'). As this dose is to be given 'twice daily', the TDD will be $256 \times 2 = 512$ mg.

If using a 125 mg/5 mL suspension, it would be appropriate to give this in four divided doses:

512 mg = 20.48 mL cefradine (cephradine) 125 mg/5 mL suspension

So the dose is: $\dfrac{20.48}{4}$ = 5.12 mL (5 ml) FOUR times a day

CALCULATING DRUG DOSAGES

There are several ways of solving this type of calculation. It is best to learn one way and stick to it.

The easiest way is by proportion: what you do to one side of an equation, do the same to the other side. The 'ONE unit' rule described in Chapter 1 'First principles' will be used here.

Also, when what you've got and what you want are in different units, you need to convert everything to the same units. When converting to the same units, it is best to convert to whole numbers to avoid decimal points, as fewer mistakes are then made. If possible, it is a good idea to convert everything to the units of the answer.

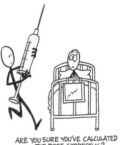

ARE YOU SURE YOU'VE CALCULATED THE DOSE CORRECTLY?

WORKED EXAMPLE

You need to give a patient 125 micrograms of digoxin orally. You have digoxin elixir 50 micrograms/mL supplied with a dropper pipette. How much do you need to draw up?

Before we continue with the calculation, we will try to estimate our answer. This is only really possible with such simple calculations.

We have: 50 micrograms in 1 mL
So: 100 micrograms in 2 mL   (by doubling)
It follows: 150 micrograms in 3 mL   (1 mL + 2 mL)
From this: 125 micrograms would be within the range 2–3 mL.

STEP ONE
Write down what you have: 50 micrograms in 1 mL

STEP TWO
Calculate how much ONE unit is of what you have, i.e.:

$$50 \text{ micrograms in 1 mL}$$

$$1 \text{ microgram} = \frac{1}{50} \text{mL}$$

This is the 'ONE unit' rule.

STEP THREE

You need to know how much digoxin to draw up for 125 micrograms, therefore multiply the amount from Step Two by 125:

$$125 \text{ micrograms} = \frac{1}{50} \times 125 = 2.5 \text{mL}$$

ANSWER: You will need to draw up 2.5 mL of digoxin.

This correlates with our estimation of our answer; 2.5 mL is within the range 2 to 3 mL. In fact, we could have easily worked out the answer exactly from our estimations.

From the above, a formula can be derived to calculate drug dosages:

$$\frac{\text{amount you want}}{\text{amount you've got}} \times \text{volume it's in}$$

This formula should be familiar as this is the one universally taught for calculating doses. Remember care must be taken when using any formula – ensure that numbers are entered and calculated correctly. From the above example:

$$\text{amount you want} = 125 \text{ micrograms}$$
$$\text{amount you've got} = 50 \text{ micrograms}$$
$$\text{volume it's in} = 1 \text{ mL}$$

Substitute the numbers in the formula:

$$\frac{125}{50} \times 1 = 2.5 \text{mL}$$

ANSWER: You will need to draw up 2.5 mL of digoxin.

You can apply this method to whatever type of calculation you want.

TIP BOX
There are several ways of solving these types of calculation. It is best to learn one way and stick to it.

The following case report illustrates the importance of ensuring that your calculations are right.

A PROBLEM WITH A DECIMAL POINT

Case report

A female baby, born seven weeks prematurely, died at 28 hours old when a junior doctor miscalculated a dose of intravenous morphine, resulting in the administration of a 100-times overdose. The doctor is reported to have worked out the dose on a piece of paper and then checked it on a calculator but the decimal point was inserted in the wrong place and 15 instead of 0.15 milligrams was prescribed. The dose was then prepared and handed to the senior registrar who administered it without double-checking the calculation and, despite treatment with naloxone, the baby died 55 minutes later.

Taken from: *Pharmacy in Practice* 1997; **7**: 368–9.

The following two cases illustrate the importance of checking numbers before administration.

BE ALERT TO HIGH NUMBERS OF DOSE UNITS

Case report

Case One

A male patient was prescribed a stat dose of 2g amiodarone for conversion of atrial fibrillation. Although it is still not known whether this dose was chosen deliberately or prescribed in error, there is evidence to support the use of a 2g oral regimen. What concerned the reporting hospital was that the nurse administered 10 × 200mg tablets to the patient without any reference or confirmation that this was indeed what was intended. This use of amiodarone is at present outside the product licence and would not have been described in any of the literature available on the ward.

The patient subsequently died, but at the time of writing no causal effect from this high dose of amiodarone had been established.

Case Two

A female patient aged approximately 65 years was prescribed 2,500 units of dalteparin sodium subcutaneously once a day as part of the DVT prophylaxis protocol. The prescribed dose was misread and two nurses checking each other gave five pre-filled syringes, i.e. 25,000 units, to the patient in error. So much heparin was required that another patient's supply had to be used as well and the error came to light when the ward made a request to pharmacy for 25,000 unit doses of dalteparin. When the error was discovered the patient's coagulation status was checked immediately and she fortunately came to no harm.

Comment

It seems inconceivable that such high numbers of dose units could be administered to patients without the nurses involved at least querying that something might be wrong.

Taken from: *Pharmacy in Practice* 2001; **6**: 194.

PROBLEMS

Question 13   You need to give 1 g of erythromycin orally. You have erythromycin suspension 250 mg in 5 mL.

How much of the suspension do you need to give?

Question 14   You need to give a patient 62.5 micrograms of digoxin orally. You have digoxin liquid containing 50 micrograms/mL.

How much do you need to draw up?

Question 15   If Oramorph® concentrate 100 mg/5 ml is used to give a dose of 60 mg for breakthrough pain, what volume is required?

Question 16   You have pethidine injection 100 mg in 2 mL. The patient is prescribed 75 mg.

How much do you draw up?

Question 17   You need to give ranitidine liquid at a dose of 2 mg/kg to a 9-year-old child weighing 23 kg.

You have a 150 mg in 10 mL liquid. How much do you need to give for each dose?

Question 18   You need to give a dose of trimethoprim suspension to a child weighing 18.45 kg at a dose of 4 mg/kg. You have trimethoprim suspension 50 mg in 5 mL.

What dose do you need to give and how much of the suspension do you need?

Question 19   Ciclosporin (cyclosporin) has been prescribed to treat a patient with severe rheumatoid arthritis. The oral dose is 2.5 mg/kg daily in two divided doses. The patient weighs 68 kg. Ciclosporin (cyclosporine) is available in 10 mg, 25 mg, 50 mg and 100 mg capsules. What dose is required and which strength of capsules would you need to give?

Question 20   You need to give aciclovir (acyclovir) as an infusion at a dose of 5 mg/kg every 8 hours. The patient weighs 76 kg and aciclovir (acyclovir) is available as 250 mg vials. How many vials do you need for each dose?

Question 21   A 50 kg woman is prescribed aminophylline as an infusion at a dose of 0.5 mg/kg/hour.

Aminophylline injection comes as 250 mg in 10 mL ampoules.

How much is required if the infusion is to run for 12 hours?

Question 22   You need to prepare an infusion of co-trimoxazole at a dose of 120 mg/kg/day in four divided doses for a patient weighing 68 kg.

Co-trimoxazole is available as 5 mL ampoules at a strength of 96 mg/mL.

i)   What volume of co-trimoxazole do you need for each dose?

ii)   How many ampoules do you need for each dose?

iii) How many ampoules do you need for 24 hours?

iv) Before administration, co-trimoxazole must be diluted further: 1 ampoule diluted to 125 mL. Therefore in what volume should each dose be given in? Round this up to the nearest commercially available bag size, i.e. 50 mL, 100 mL, 250 mL, 500 mL or 1 litre.

Answers can be found on page 190.

DISPLACEMENT VALUES OR VOLUMES

Dry powder injections need to be reconstituted with a diluent before they are used. Sometimes the final volume of the injection will be greater than the volume of liquid that was added to the powder. This volume difference is called the injection's displacement value.

What is displacement?

If you take ordinary salt and dissolve it in some water, the resultant solution will have a greater volume than before. The salt appears to 'displace' some water increasing the volume.

Antibiotic suspensions are good examples to illustrate displacement.

For example, to make up 100 mL of amoxicillin (amoxycillin) suspension, only 68 mL of water needs to be added. The amoxicillin (amoxycillin) powder must therefore displace 32 mL of water, i.e. $100 - 68 = 32$ mL.

Is displacement important in medicine?

For most patients this does not matter because the whole vial is administered. However it can be very important when you want to give a dose that is less than the total contents of the vial – a frequent occurrence in paediatrics and neonatology.

The volume of the final solution must be considered when calculating the amount to withdraw from the vial. The total volume may be increased significantly and, if this is not taken into account, significant errors in dosage may occur, especially when small doses are involved as with neonates. For example:

Cefotaxime at a dose of 50 mg/kg 12-hourly
for a baby weighing 3.6 kg.

Therefore dose required = $50 \times 3.6 = 180$ mg

Displacement volume for cefotaxime = 0.2 mL for a 500 mg vial.

Therefore you need to add 1.8 mL $(2 - 0.2)$ water for injection to give a final concentration of:

500 mg in 2 mL

Thus the required dose in mL is:

$$180 \text{ mg} = \frac{2}{500} \times 180 = 0.72 \text{mL}$$

If the displacement volume is not taken into account, then you will have:

500 mg in 2.2 mL (2 mL + 0.2 mL displacement volume)

You worked out earlier that the dose required is 180 mg and this is equal to 0.72 mL (assuming you have 500 mg in 2 mL). But now 0.72 mL contains:

$$\frac{500}{2.2} \times 0.72 = 164 \text{mg}$$

(since the actual volume you have is 2.2 mL and **not** 2 mL).

Thus if the displacement volume is not taken into account, then the amount drawn up is 164 mg and not 180 mg as required.

Displacement values will depend on the medicine, the manufacturer and its strength. Information on a medicine's displacement value is usually stated in the relevant drug information sheets, in paediatric dosage books, or can be obtained from your Pharmacy Department.

Calculating doses using displacement volumes:

volume to be added = diluent volume – displacement volume

For example, for **benzylpenicillin**:

Dose required = 450 mg
Displacement volume = 0.4 mL per 600 mg vial
Total diluted volume = 5 mL
Volume of diluent to be added = 5 – 0.4 = 4.6 mL
Final concentration = 120 mg/mL
Volume required to deliver 450 mg dose = 3.75 mL

PROBLEMS

Work out the following dosages, not forgetting to take into account displacement values if necessary.

Question 23   You need to give a 4-month-old child 350 mg ceftriaxone IV daily.

You have a 1 g vial that needs to be reconstituted to 10 mL with Water for Injections. Displacement value = 0.8 mL for 1 g.

i) Taking into account displacement volumes, what volume should you add to the vial?

ii) How much do you need to draw up for a 350 mg dose?

Question 24 You need to give cefotaxime IV to a 5-year-old child weighing 18 kg at a dose of 150 mg/kg/day in four divided doses.

You have a 1 g vial that needs to be reconstituted to 4 mL with Water for Injections. Displacement value = 0.5 mL for 1 g.

i) Taking into account displacement volumes, what volume should you add to the vial?

ii) How much do you need to draw up for each dose?

Question 25 You need to give flucloxacillin IV to an 8-year-old child weighing 19.6 kg. The dose is 12.5 mg/kg four times a day.

You have a 250 mg vial that needs to be reconstituted to 5 mL with Water for Injections. Displacement value = 0.2 mL for 250 mg.

i) Taking into account displacement volumes, what volume should you add to the vial?

ii) How much do you need to draw up for each dose?

Answers can be found on page 193.

7 MOLES AND MILLIMOLES

OBJECTIVES

At the end of this chapter, you should be familiar with the following:

- Moles and millimoles
- Millimoles and micromoles
- Calculations involving moles and millimoles
    - Conversion of milligrams to millimoles
    - Conversion of percentage strength (% w/v) to millimoles
- Molar solutions and molarity

KEY POINTS

Moles

- The **mole** is a unit used by chemists to count atoms and molecules.
- A mole of any substance is the amount that contains the same number of particles of the substance as there are atoms in $12\,g$ of carbon (C^{12}) – known as Avogadro's number.
- For elements or atoms:

    one mole = the **atomic mass** in grams
- For molecules:

    one mole = the **molecular mass** in grams

Millimoles

- Moles are too big for everyday use, so the unit **millimoles** is used.
- One millimole is equal to one-thousandth of a mole.
- If one mole is the atomic mass or molecular mass in grams, it follows that:

    one **millimole** = the **atomic mass** or **molecular mass** in **milligrams**

Conversion of Milligrams (mg) to Millimoles (mmol)
mg/mL to millimoles

$$\text{total number of millimoles} = \frac{\text{strength in mg/mL}}{\text{mg of substance containing 1 mmol}} \times \text{volume (in mL)}$$

Conversion of percentage strength (% w/v) to millimoles

$$\text{total number of mmol} = \frac{\text{percentage strength (\% w/v)}}{\text{mg of substance containing 1 mmol}} \times 10 \times \text{volume (mL)}$$

Molar Solutions and Molarity

- Molarity is a term used in chemistry to describe concentrations:

When **one mole** of a substance is dissolved in **one litre** of solution, it is known as a **one molar (1 M)** solution.

- A one molar (1 M) solution has one mole of the substance dissolved in each litre of solution (equivalent to 1 mmol per mL).
- If 2 moles of a substance are made up to 1 litre (or 1 mole to 500 mL), the solution is said to be a 2 M solution.

INTRODUCTION

Daily references may be made to moles and millimoles in relation to electrolyte levels, blood glucose, serum creatinine or other blood results with regard to patients. These are measurements carried out by chemical pathology and the units used are usually millimoles or micromoles. The millimole unit is also encountered with infusions when electrolytes have been added.

For example:

Mr J. Brown   Sodium = 138 mmol/L

'The infusion contains 20 mmol potassium chloride.'

Before you can interpret such results or amounts, you will need to be familiar with this rather confusing unit: the mole.

This section will explain what moles and millimoles are, and how to do calculations involving millimoles.

WHAT ARE MOLES AND MILLIMOLES?

It is important to know what moles and millimoles are and how they are derived. However, the concept of moles and millimoles is difficult to explain and to understand; you need to be familiar with basic chemistry.

Chemists are concerned with atoms, ions and molecules. These are too small to be counted individually, so the mole is the unit used by chemists to make counting and measuring a lot easier.

So what is a mole? Just as the word 'dozen' represents the number 12, the mole also represents a number – 6×10^{23}. This number can represent atoms, ions or molecules, e.g. 1 mole of atoms is 6×10^{23} atoms. The mole is the SI unit for the amount of a substance and so one mole also represents the relative atomic, molecular or ionic mass in grams.

The atomic mass of potassium is 39; so 1 mole of potassium has a mass of 39 g (which is the same as saying that 6×10^{23} atoms of potassium have a total mass of 39 g).

Similarly, the molecular weight of sodium chloride is 58.5; therefore a mole of sodium chloride has a mass of 58.5 g and 2 moles of sodium chloride have a mass of 117 g (2×58.5).

Chemists are not the only the people who 'count by weighing'. Bank clerks use the same idea when they count coins by weighing them. For example, one hundred 1p coins weigh 356 g; it is quicker to weigh 356 g of 1p coins than to count a hundred coins.

Now consider a single molecule of sodium chloride (NaCl) which consists of one sodium ion (Na^+) and one chloride ion (Cl^-).

$$NaCl \qquad = \text{molecule}$$

$$Na+ \quad Cl- \qquad = \text{ions}$$

Since moles can refer to ions as well as molecules, it can be seen that one mole of sodium chloride contains one mole of sodium ions and one mole of chloride ions. From tables (see the end of this section), the relative ionic masses are:

sodium (Na) 23
chloride (Cl) 35.5

The molecular mass is the sum of the ionic masses:

sodium (Na) 23
chloride (Cl) <u>35.5</u>
<u>58.5</u> = molecular mass of NaCl

So we can say that:

1 mole of sodium ion weighs 23 g;
1 mole of chloride ion weighs 35.5 g;
1 mole of sodium chloride weighs 58.5 g

Next consider calcium chloride ($CaCl_2$). Each molecule consists of **one** calcium ion and **two** chloride ions. The '2' after the 'Cl' means **two** ions of chlorine:

$$CaCl_2 \qquad = \text{molecule}$$

$$Ca^{2+} \quad Cl^- + Cl^- \qquad = \text{ions}$$

The molecular mass of calcium chloride is 147. The reason why the molecular mass does not always equal the sum of the atomic masses of the individual ions is because water forms a part of each calcium chloride molecule.

The molecule is actually $CaCl_2 \cdot 2H_2O$. From the molecular formula and knowledge of the atomic weights it can be seen that calcium chloride contains:

1 mole of Ca = 40 g
2 moles of Cl = 71 g
2 moles of H_2O, each mole of water = 18 g; 2 × 18 = 36 g

So adding everything together:

$$(40 + 71 + 36) = 147$$

i.e. the mass of 1 mole $CaCl_2$ is 147 g.

TABLE 7.1 ATOMIC AND MOLECULAR MASS	
ATOM/MOLECULE	**MASS**
Calcium (Ca)	40
Calcium chloride	147
Calcium gluconate	448.5
Carbon (C)	12
Chloride (Cl)	35.5
Dextrose/glucose	180
Hydrogen (H)	1
Magnesium (Mg)	24
Magnesium chloride	203
Magnesium sulphate	246.5
Oxygen (O)	16
Potassium (K)	39
Potassium chloride	74.5
Sodium (Na)	23
Sodium bicarbonate	84
Sodium chloride	58.5
Sodium citrate	294
Sodium phosphate	358
Water (H_2O)	18

MILLIMOLES AND MICROMOLES

Moles are, however, too big for everyday use in medicine, so millimoles and micromoles are used.

> One millimole is equal to one-thousandth of a mole
>
> One micromole is equal to one-thousandth of a millimole

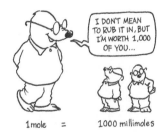

I DON'T MEAN TO RUB IT IN, BUT I'M WORTH 1,000 OF YOU...

1 mole = 1000 millimoles

It follows that:

> 1 mole contains 1,000 millimoles (mmol)
> 1 millimole contains 1,000 micromoles (mcmol)

So, in the above explanation, you can substitute millimoles for moles and milligrams for grams. For our purposes:

Sodium chloride	would give ➝	sodium	+	chloride
1 **mole** or		1 **mole** or		1 **mole** or
1 **millimole**		1 **millimole**		1 **millimole**
58.5 g or		23 g or		
	35.5 g or			
58.5 mg		23 mg		
	35.5 mg			

The following are examples and problems to see if you understand the concept of millimoles. It is unlikely that you will encounter these types of calculations on the ward, but it is useful to know how they are done and they can be used for reference if necessary.

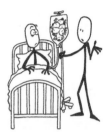

WELL, YES... THE DRUG CHART **DID** SAY 100 millimoles/litre BUT I COULD ONLY SQUEEZE IN 10!

CALCULATIONS INVOLVING MOLES AND MILLIMOLES

Conversion of milligrams (mg) to millimoles (mmol)

Sometimes it may be necessary to calculate the number of millimoles in an infusion or injection or to convert mg/litre to mmol/litre.

WORKED EXAMPLE

How many millimoles of sodium are there in a 500 mL infusion containing 1.8 mg/mL sodium chloride?

STEP ONE

As already stated: 1 millimole of sodium chloride yields 1 millimole of sodium. So it follows that the amount (in milligrams) equal to 1 millimole of sodium chloride will give 1 millimole of sodium.

In this case, calculate the total amount (in milligrams) of sodium chloride and convert this to millimoles to find out the number of millimoles of sodium.

STEP TWO

Calculate the total amount of sodium chloride.
You have an infusion containing 1.8 mg/mL.
Therefore in 500 mL, you have:

$$1.8 \times 500 = 900 \text{ mg sodium chloride}$$

STEP THREE

From tables: molecular mass of sodium chloride (NaCl) = 58.5.

So 1 millimole of sodium chloride (NaCl) will weigh 58.5 mg and this amount will give 1 millimole of sodium (Na).

STEP FOUR

Next calculate the number of millimoles in the infusion. First work out the number of millimoles for 1 mg of sodium chloride, and then the number for the total amount.

58.5 mg sodium chloride will give 1 millimole of sodium.

1 mg will give $\dfrac{1}{58.5}$ millimoles of sodium.

So, 900 mg will give $\dfrac{1}{58.5} \times 900 = 15.38$ mmol (or 15 mmol approx.)

ANSWER: There are 15.4 mmol (approximately 15 mmol) of sodium in a 500 mL infusion containing 1.8 mg/mL sodium chloride.

Alternatively, a formula can be used:

total number of millimoles $= \dfrac{\text{mg/mL}}{\text{mg of substance containing 1 mmol}} \times \text{volume(mL)}$

where, in this case

mg/mL $= 1.8$

mg of substance containing 1 mmol $= 58.5$

volume (mL) $= 500$

Substituting the numbers in the formula:

$\dfrac{1.8}{58.5}$ mmol $\times 500 = 15.38$ mmol (or 15 mmol approx.)

ANSWER: There are 15.4 mmol (approximately 15 mmol) of sodium in a 500 mL infusion containing 1.8 mg/mL sodium chloride.

PROBLEMS

Question 1   How many millimoles of sodium are there in a 500 mL infusion containing 27 mg/mL sodium chloride? (MM sodium chloride = 58.5)

Question 2   How many millimoles of sodium are there in a 10 mL ampoule containing 300 mg/mL sodium chloride? (MM sodium chloride = 58.5)

Question 3   How many millimoles of sodium, potassium and chloride are there in a 500 mL infusion containing 9 mg/mL sodium chloride and potassium chloride 3 mg/mL? (MM sodium chloride = 58.5; MW potassium chloride = 74.5)

Question 4   How many millimoles of glucose are there in a 1 litre infusion containing 50 g/litre glucose? (MM glucose = 180)

Answers can be found on page 195.

Conversion of percentage strength (% w/v) to millimoles

Sometimes it may be necessary to convert percentage strength to the number of millimoles. This is very similar to the previous example. All you need to do is to convert the percentage strength to the number of milligrams in the required volume, then follow the steps as before.

> **WORKED EXAMPLE**
>
> How many millimoles of sodium are in 1 litre of sodium chloride 0.9% infusion?
>
> *STEP ONE*
>
> We know that 1 millimole of sodium chloride will give 1 millimole of sodium.
>
> So, the amount (in milligrams) equal to 1 millimole of sodium chloride will give 1 millimole of sodium.
>
> *STEP TWO*
>
> To calculate the number of milligrams in 1 millimole of sodium chloride, either refer to tables or work from first principles using atomic masses.
>
> From tables: molecular mass of sodium chloride (NaCl) = 58.5.
>
> So 1 millimole of sodium chloride (NaCl) will weigh 58.5 mg and this amount will give 1 millimole of sodium (Na).
>
> *STEP THREE*
>
> Calculate the total amount of sodium chloride present:
>
> $$0.9\% = 0.9\,g \text{ in } 100\,mL$$
> $$= 900\,mg \text{ in } 100\,mL$$
>
> Thus in a 1 litre (1,000 mL) infusion, the amount is:
>
> $$\frac{900}{100} \times 1,000 = 9,000\,mg \text{ or } 9\,g$$
>
> *STEP FOUR*
>
> From Step Two, it was found that:
>
> 58.5 mg sodium chloride will give 1 millimole of sodium.
>
> So it follows that:
>
> 1 mg of sodium chloride will give $\dfrac{1}{58.5}$ millimoles of sodium.
>
> So, 9,000 mg sodium chloride will give
>
> $$\frac{1}{58.5} \times 9,000 = 153.8 \text{ (154) mmol of sodium}$$

ANSWER: 1 litre of sodium chloride 0.9% infusion contains 154 mmol of sodium (approx.).

A formula can be devised:

$$mmol = \frac{\text{percentage strength (\% w/v)}}{\text{mg of substance containing 1 mmol}} \times 10 \times \text{volume (mL)}$$

In this example:

$$\text{percentage strength (\% w/v)} = 0.9$$
$$\text{mg of substance containing 1 mmol} = 58.5$$
$$\text{volume (mL)} = 1,000$$

Then 10 simply converts percentage strength (g/100 mL) to mg/mL (everything in the same units).

Substituting the numbers in the formula:

$$\frac{0.9}{58.5} \times 10 \times 1,000 = 153.8 \, (154) \, mmol \text{ of sodium}$$

ANSWER: 1 litre of sodium chloride 0.9% infusion contains 154 mmol of sodium (approx.).

PROBLEMS

Question 5   How many millimoles of sodium are there in a 1 litre infusion of glucose 4% and sodium chloride 0.18%? (MM sodium chloride = 58.5; glucose = 180.)

Question 6   How many millimoles of calcium and chloride are there in a 10 mL ampoule of calcium chloride 10%? (MM calcium chloride = 147)
Note: calcium chloride = $CaCl_2$

Question 7   How many millimoles of calcium are there in a 10 mL ampoule of calcium gluconate 10%? (MM calcium gluconate = 448.5)

Question 8   How many millimoles of sodium are there in a 200 mL infusion of sodium bicarbonate 8.4%? (MM sodium bicarbonate = 84)

Answers can be found on page 196.

MOLAR SOLUTIONS AND MOLARITY

Molarity is a term used in chemistry to describe concentrations. When moles of substances are dissolved in water to make solutions, the unit of concentration is molarity and the solutions are known as molar solutions.

When **one mole** of a substance is dissolved in **one litre** of solution, it is known as a **one molar (1 M)** solution. This is equivalent to 1 mmol per mL.

If 2 moles of a substance are made up to 1 litre (or 1 mole to 500 mL), the solution is said to be a two molar (2 M) solution.

WORKED EXAMPLES

If 18 g of sodium citrate is made up to 200 mL of solution, what is the molarity of the solution? (MW sodium citrate = 294).

STEP ONE
Write down the weight of one mole:

$$1 \text{ mole of sodium citrate} = 294\,g$$

STEP TWO
Calculate the number of moles for 1 g (using the 'ONE unit' rule):

$$1\,g \text{ would equal } \frac{1}{294} \text{ moles}$$

STEP THREE
Calculate the number of moles for 18 g:

$$18\,g = \frac{1}{294} \times 18 = \frac{18}{294} = 0.06 \text{ moles}$$

You therefore have 0.06 moles in 200 mL.

STEP FOUR
Convert to a molar concentration. To do this, you need to calculate the equivalent number of moles per litre (1,000 mL).
You have 0.06 moles in 200 mL:

$$1\,mL = \frac{0.06}{200} \text{ moles}$$

Therefore in 1,000 mL there are:

$$\frac{0.06}{200} \times 1,000 = 0.06 \times 5 = 0.3 \text{ moles}$$

ANSWER: If 18 g of sodium citrate is made up to 200 mL, the resulting solution would have a concentration of 0.3 M.

Alternatively, a formula can be derived:

$$\text{concentration (mol/L or M)} = \frac{\text{number of moles}}{\text{volume in litres}}$$

The *number of moles* is calculated from the weight (in g) and the molecular mass:

$$\text{moles} = \frac{\text{weight (g)}}{\text{molecular mass}}$$

To convert the volume (in mL) to *litres*, divide by 1,000:

$$\text{volume in litres} = \frac{\text{volume (mL)}}{1,000}$$

Putting these together gives the following formula:

$$\text{concentration (mol/L or M)} = \frac{\text{number of moles}}{\text{volume in litres}} = \frac{\dfrac{\text{weight (s)}}{\text{molucular mass}}}{\dfrac{\text{volume (mL)}}{1,000}}$$

Re-writing this gives:

$$\text{concentration (mol/L or M)} = \frac{\text{weight (g)} \times 1,000}{\text{molecular mass} \times \text{volume (mL)}}$$

In this example:

$$\text{weight (g)} = 18$$
$$\text{molecular mass} = 294$$
$$\text{volume (mL)} = 200$$

Substitute the figures into the formula:

$$\text{concentration} = \frac{18 \times 1,000}{294 \times 200} = 0.3 \text{ M}$$

ANSWER: If 18 g of sodium citrate is made up to 200 mL, the resulting solution would have a concentration of 0.3 M.

The calculation can also be done in reverse. For example, how many grams of sodium citrate are needed to make 100 mL of a 0.5 M solution?

STEP ONE
Write down the final concentration needed and what it signifies:

$$0.5 \text{ M} = 0.5 \text{ moles in } 1,000 \text{ mL}$$

STEP TWO
Work out the number of moles needed for the volume required. You have:

$$0.5 \text{ moles in } 1,000 \text{ mL}$$

Therefore:

$$1 \text{ mL} = \frac{0.5}{1,000} \text{ moles}$$

For 100 mL, you will need:

$$100\,mL = \frac{0.5}{1,000} \times 100 = \frac{0.5}{10} = 0.05 \text{ moles}$$

STEP THREE

Convert moles to grams. You know that 1 mole sodium citrate has a mass of 294 g.

$$1 \text{ mole} = 294\,g$$

Therefore:

$$0.05 \text{ moles} = 294 \times 0.05 = 14.7\,g$$

ANSWER: If 14.7 g of sodium citrate is made up to 100 mL, the resulting solution would have a concentration of 0.5 M.

Alternatively, a formula can be derived:

$$\text{concentration (mol/L or M)} = \frac{\text{number of moles}}{\text{volume in litres}}$$

so:

$$\text{number of moles} = \text{concentration (mol/L or M)} \times \text{volume in litres}$$

We want to go a step further and calculate a weight (in grams) instead of number of moles. The *number of moles* is calculated from the weight (in grams) and the molecular mass:

$$\text{moles} = \frac{\text{weight (g)}}{\text{molecular mass}}$$

To convert the volume (in mL) to *litres*, divide by 1,000:

$$\text{volume in litres} = \frac{\text{volume (mL)}}{1,000}$$

Putting these together gives the following formula:

$$\text{moles} = \frac{\text{weight (g)}}{\text{molecular mass}} = \text{concentration (mol/L or M)} \times \frac{\text{volume (mL)}}{1,000}$$

Re-writing this gives:

$$\text{weight (g)} = \frac{\text{concentration (mol/L or M)} \times \text{molecular mass} \times \text{final volume (mL)}}{1,000}$$

In this example:

$$\text{concentration (mol/L or M)} = 0.5$$
$$\text{molecular mass} = 294$$
$$\text{final volume (mL)} = 100$$

Substitute the figures in the formula:

$$\frac{0.5 \times 294 \times 100}{1,000} = 14.7\,g$$

ANSWER: If 14.7 g of sodium citrate is made up to 100 mL, the resulting solution would have a concentration of 0.5 M.

PROBLEMS

Question 9   If 8.4 g of sodium bicarbonate is made up to 50 mL of solution, what is the molarity of the solution? (MM sodium bicarbonate = 84)

Question 10   How many grams of sodium citrate are needed to make 250 mL of a 0.1 M solution? (MM sodium citrate = 294)

Answers can be found on page 199.

OBJECTIVES

At the end of this chapter you should be familiar with the following:

- Drip rate calculations (drops/min)
- Conversion of dosages to mL/hour
- Conversion of mL/hour back to a dose
- Calculating the length of time for IV infusions

KEY POINTS

Drip Rate Calculations (drops/min)

- In all drip rate calculations, you have to remember that you are simply converting a volume to drops (or vice versa) and hours to minutes.

$$\text{drops/min} = \frac{\text{drops/mL of the giving set} \times \text{volume of the infusion (mL)}}{\text{number of hours the infusion is to run} \times 60}$$

Giving sets

- The **standard giving set (SGS)** has a drip rate of **20 drops per mL** for clear fluids (i.e. sodium chloride, glucose) and **15 drops per mL** for blood.
- The **micro-drop giving set** or burette has a drip rate of **60 drops per mL**.

Conversion of Dosages to mL/hour

- In this type of calculation, it is best to convert the dose required to a volume in millilitres.
- Doses expressed as mcg/kg/min:

$$\text{mL/hour} = \frac{\text{volume to be infused} \times \text{dose} \times \text{weight} \times 60}{\text{amount if drug} \times 1,000}$$

60 converts minutes to hours.
1,000 converts mcg to mg.

- If doses are expressed in milligrams, then there is no need to divide by 1,000.
- If doses are expressed as a total dose, i.e. dose/min, there is no need to multiply by the patient's weight.

Conversion of mL/hour Back to a Dose

- Sometimes it may be necessary to convert *mL/hour* back to the dose in *mg/min* or *mcg/min* and *mg/kg/min* or *mcg/kg/min*.

$$\text{mcg/kg/min} = \frac{\text{rate (mL/hour)} \times \text{amount of drug} \times 1,000}{\text{weight (kg)} \times \text{volume (mL)} \times 60}$$

1,000 converts mcg to mg.
60 converts minutes to hours.

- If doses are expressed in terms of milligrams, then there is no need to multiply by 1,000.
- If doses are expressed as a total dose, i.e. dose/min, there is no need to divide by the patient's weight.

Calculating the Length of Time for IV Infusions

- Sometimes it may be necessary to calculate the number of hours an infusion should run at a specified rate. Also, it is a good way of checking your calculated drip rate for an infusion.

Manually controlled infusions

$$\text{number of hours the infusion is to run} = \frac{\text{volume of the infusion}}{\text{rate (drops/min)} \times 60} \times \text{drip rate of giving set}$$

Infusion or syringe pumps

$$\text{number of hours the infusion is to run} = \frac{\text{volume of the infusion}}{\text{rate (mL/hour)}}$$

INTRODUCTION

With infusions, there are two types of infusion rate calculations to be considered: those involving **drops/min** and those involving **mL/hour**.

The first (drops/min) is mainly encountered when infusions are given under gravity as with fluid replacement. The second (mL/hour) is encountered when infusions have to be given accurately or in small volumes using infusion or syringe pumps – particularly if drugs have to be given as infusions.

DRIP RATE CALCULATIONS (drops/min)

To set up a manually controlled infusion accurately, you need to be able to count the number of drops per minute. To do this, you have to calculate the volume to be infused in terms of drops. This in turn depends upon the giving or administration set being used.

Giving sets

There are two giving sets:

- The **standard giving set (SGS)** has a drip rate of **20 drops per mL** for clear fluids (i.e. sodium chloride, glucose) and **15 drops per mL** for blood.
- The **micro-drop giving set** or burette has a drip rate of **60 drops per mL**.

The drip rate of the giving set is always written on the wrapper if you are not sure.

In all drip rate calculations, you have to remember that you are simply converting a volume to drops (or vice versa) and hours to minutes.

WORKED EXAMPLE

1 litre of sodium chloride 0.9% ('normal saline') is to be given over 8 hours: what drip rate is required using a standard giving set (SGS), 20 drops/mL?

STEP ONE

First convert the volume to a number of drops. To do this, multiply the volume of the infusion by the number of 'drops per mL' for the giving set, i.e.

$$1 \text{ litre} = 1{,}000 \text{ mL, so it will be}$$
$$1{,}000 \times 20 = 20{,}000 \text{ drops}$$

You have just calculated the number of drops to be infused.

STEP TWO

Next convert hours to minutes by multiplying the number of hours over which the infusion is to be given by 60 (60 minutes = 1 hour).

$$8 \text{ hours} = 8 \times 60 = 480 \text{ minutes}$$

Now everything has been converted in terms of drops and minutes, i.e. what you want for your final answer.

If the infusion is being given over a period of minutes, then obviously there is no need to convert from hours to minutes.

STEP THREE

Write down what you have just calculated, i.e. the total number of drops to be given over how many minutes.

$$20{,}000 \text{ drops to be given over 480 minutes}$$

STEP FOUR

Calculate the number of drops per minute by dividing the number of drops by the number of minutes:

$$\frac{20{,}000}{480} = 41.67 \text{ drops/min}$$

Since it is impossible to have part of a drop, round up or down to the nearest whole number:

$$41.67 \approx 42 \text{ drops/min}$$

ANSWER: To give a litre (1,000 mL) of sodium chloride 0.9% ('normal saline') over 8 hours using a standard giving set (20 drops/mL), the rate will have to be 42 drops/min.

A formula can be used:

$$\text{drops/min} = \frac{\text{drops/mL of the giving set} \times \text{volume of the infusion (mL)}}{\text{number of hours the infusion is to run} \times 60}$$

where in this case:

drops/mL of the giving set = 20 drops/mL (SGS)

volume of the infusion (in mL) = 1,000 mL

number of hours the infusion is to run = 8 hours

60 = number of minutes in an hour (converts hours to minutes)

Substituting the numbers into the formula:

$$\frac{20 \times 1,000}{8 \times 60} = 41.67 \text{ drops/min (42 drops/min, approx.)}$$

ANSWER: To give a litre (1,000 mL) of sodium chloride 0.9% ('normal saline') over 8 hours using a standard giving set (20 drops/mL), the rate will have to be 42 drops/min .

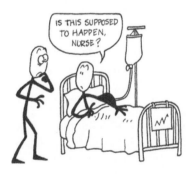

PROBLEMS

Work out the drip rates for the following infusions:

Question 1   500 mL of sodium chloride 0.9% over 6 hours

Question 2   1 litre of glucose 4% and sodium chloride 0.18% over 12 hours

Question 3   1 unit of blood (500 mL) over 6 hours

Answers can be found on page 201.

CONVERSION OF DOSAGES TO mL/hour

Dosages can be expressed in various ways: *mg/min* or *mcg/min* and *mg/kg/min* or *mcg/kg/min*; and it may be necessary to convert to *mL/hour* (when using infusion pumps).

The following example shows the various steps in this type of calculation, and this can be adapted for any dosage to infusion rate calculation.

WORKED EXAMPLE

You have an infusion of dopamine 800 mg in 500 mL. The dose required is 2 mcg/kg/min for a patient weighing 68 kg. What is the rate in mL/hour?

STEP ONE

When doing this type of calculation, you need to convert the dose required to a volume in mL and minutes to hours.

STEP TWO

First calculate the dose required:

$$\text{dose required} = \text{patient's weight} \times \text{dose prescribed}$$
$$= 68 \times 2 = 136 \text{ mcg/min}$$

If the dose is given as a total dose and not on a weight basis, then miss out this step.

STEP THREE

The dose is 136 mcg/min. The final answer needs to be in terms of hours, so multiply by 60 to convert minutes into hours:

$$136 \times 60 = 8,160 \text{ mcg/hour}$$

Convert mcg to mg by dividing by 1,000:

$$\frac{8,160}{1,000} = 8.16 \text{ mg/hour}$$

STEP FOUR

The next step is to calculate the volume for the dose required.
Calculate the volume for 1 mg of drug:
You have: 800 mg in 500 mL:

$$1 \text{ mg} = \frac{500}{800} = 0.625 \text{ mL}$$

STEP FIVE

Thus for the dose of 8.16 mg, the volume is equal to:

$$8.16 \text{ mg} = 0.625 \times 8.16 = 5.1 \text{ mL/hour}$$

ANSWER: The rate required is 5.1 mL/hour.

A formula can be derived:

$$mL/hour = \frac{\text{volume to be infused} \times \text{dose} \times \text{weight} \times 60}{\text{amount of drug} \times 1{,}000}$$

In this case:

> total volume to be infused = 500 mL
> total amount of drug (mg) = 800 mg
> dose = 2 mcg/kg/min
> patient's weight = 68 kg
> 60 converts minutes to hours
> 1,000 converts mcg to mg

Substituting the numbers into the formula:

$$\frac{500 \times 2 \times 68 \times 60}{800 \times 1{,}000} = 5.1 \text{ mL/hour}$$

ANSWER: The rate required is 5.1 mL/hour.

If the dose is given as a total dose and not on a weight basis, then the patient's weight is not needed.

$$mL/hour = \frac{\text{volume to be infused} \times \text{dose} \times 60}{\text{amount of drug} \times 1{,}000}$$

Note:
- If doses are expressed in terms of milligrams, then there is no need to divide by 1,000.
- If doses are expressed as a total dose, i.e. dose/min, there is no need to multiply by the patient's weight.

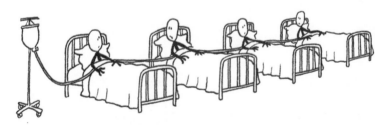

I KNOW THEY'RE SUPPOSED TO CUT COSTS,
BUT THIS IS RIDICULOUS!

TABLE OF INFUSION RATES (ML/HOUR)

	MINUTES					HOURS										
Time / Vol	10	15	20	30	40	1	2	3	4	6	8	10	12	16	18	24
10 mL	60	40	30	20												
20 mL	120	80	60	40												
30 mL				60												
40 mL				80	60	40										
50 mL				100	75	50										
60 mL				120	90	60										
80 mL				160	120	80										
100 mL				200	150	100	50	33	25	17						
125 mL				250	188	125	63	42	31	21						
150 mL				300	225	150	75	50	38	25						
200 mL				400	300	200	100	67	50	33	25	20	17	13	11	8
250 mL							125	83	63	42	31	25	21	16	14	10
500 mL									125	83	63	50	42	31	28	21
1000 mL									250	167	125	100	83	63	56	42

Rates given in the table have been rounded up or down to give whole numbers.

How to use the table

If you need to give a 250 mL infusion over 8 hours, then to find the infusion rate (mL/hour) go down the left-hand (Vol) column until you reach 250 mL; then go along the top (Time) line until you reach 8 (for 8 hours). Then read off the corresponding infusion rate (mL/hour). In this case it is 31 mL/hour.

PROBLEMS

Question 4   You have a 500 mL infusion containing 50 mg nitroglycerin. A dose of 10 mcg/min is required.

What is the rate in mL/hour?

Question 5   You are asked to give 500 mL of lidocaine (lignocaine) 0.2% in glucose at a rate of 2 mg/min.

What is the rate in mL/hour?

Question 6   You have an infusion of dopamine 800 mg in 500 mL. The dose required is 3 mcg/kg/min for a patient weighing 80 kg.

What is the rate in mL/hour?

Question 7   A patient with chronic obstructive pulmonary disease (COPD) is to have a continuous infusion of aminophylline. The patient weighs 63 kg and the dose to be given is 0.5 mg/kg/hour over 12 hours.

Aminophylline injection comes as 250 mg in 10 mL ampoules and should be given in a 500 mL infusion bag.

(i)   What dose and volume of aminophylline are required?

(ii) What is the rate in mL/hour?

Question 8   You need to give aciclovir (acyclovir) as an infusion at a dose of 5 mg/kg every 8 hours. The patient weighs 86 kg and aciclovir (acyclovir) is available as 500 mg vials. Each vial needs to be reconstituted with 20 mL Water for Injection and diluted further to 100 mL. The infusion should be given over 60 minutes.

(i)   What dose and volume of aciclovir (acyclovir) are required for one dose?

(ii) What is the rate in mL/hour for each dose?

Question 9   Glyceryl trinitrate is to be given at a rate of 150 mcg/min. You have an infusion of 50 mg in 50 mL glucose 5%.

What is the rate in mL/hour?

Question 10 You have an infusion of dobutamine 250 mg in 50 mL. The dose required is 6 mcg/kg/min and the patient weighs 75 kg.

What is the rate in mL/hour?

Question 11 A patient with MRSA is prescribed IV vancomycin 1 g every 24 hours. After reconstitution a 500 mg vial of vancomycin should be diluted with infusion fluid to 5 mg/mL.

    (i) What is the minimum volume (ml) of infusion fluid that 1 g vancomycin can be administered in? (Round this to the nearest commercially available bag size, i.e. 50 mL, 100 mL, 250 mL, 500 mL or 1,000 mL.)

    (ii) The rate of administration not exceed 10 mg/min. Over how many minutes should the infusion be given?

    (iii) What is the rate in mL/hour?

Question 12 You are asked to give an infusion of dobutamine to a patient weighing 73 kg at a dose of 5 mcg/kg/min. You have an infusion of 500 mL sodium chloride 0.9% containing 250 mg of dobutamine.

    (i) What is the dose required (mcg/min)?

    (ii) What is the concentration (mcg/mL) of dobutamine?

    (iii) What is the rate in mL/hour?

Question 13 You are asked to give an infusion of isosorbide dinitrate 50 mg in 500 mL of glucose 5% at a rate of 2 mg/hour.

    (i) What is the rate in mL/hour?

The rate is then changed to 5 mg/hour.

    (ii) What is the new rate in mL/hour?

Answers can be found on page 202.

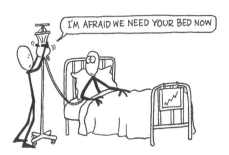

INCREASING THE INFUSION RATE

CONVERSION OF mL/hour BACK TO A DOSE

Sometimes it may be necessary to convert *mL/hour* back to the dose: *mg/min* or *mcg/min* and *mg/kg/min* or *mcg/kg/min*.

    For example, you may need to check that an infusion pump is giving the correct dose. Nurses changing shifts, especially on the critical care wards, must check that the pumps are set correctly at the beginning of each shift.

WORKED EXAMPLE

An infusion pump containing 250 mg dobutamine in 50 mL is running at a rate of 3.5 mL/hour. Convert this to mcg/kg/min to check that the pump is set correctly. (Patient's weight = 73 kg)

STEP ONE

In this type of calculation, convert the volume being given to the amount of drug, and then work out the amount of drug being given per minute or per kilogram of the patient's weight.

STEP TWO

You have 250 mg of dobutamine in 50 mL.

First it is necessary to work out the amount in 1 mL:

$$250 \text{ mg in } 50 \text{ mL}$$

$$1 \text{ mL} = \frac{250}{50} \text{ mg} = 5 \text{ mg (using the 'ONE unit' rule)}$$

STEP THREE

The rate at which the pump is running is 3.5 mL/hour. You have just worked out the amount in 1 mL (Step Two)

$$3.5 \text{ mL/hour} = 5 \times 3.5 = 17.5 \text{ mg/hour}$$

Now convert the rate (mL/hour) to the amount of drug being given over an hour.

STEP FOUR

The question asks for the dose in *mcg/kg/m* so convert milligrams to micrograms by multiplying by 1,000:

$$17.5 \times 1,000 = 17,500 \text{ mcg/hour}$$

STEP FIVE

Now calculate the rate per minute by dividing by 60 (converts hours to minutes):

$$\frac{17,500}{60} = 291.67 \text{ mcg/min}$$

STEP SIX

The final step in the calculation is to work out the rate according to the patient's weight (73 kg). (If the dose is not given in terms of the patient's weight, then miss out this final step.)

$$\frac{291.67}{73} = 3.99 \text{ mcg/kg/min}$$

This can be rounded up to 4 mcg/kg/min.

Now check your answer against the dose written on the drug chart to see if the pump is delivering the correct dose. If your answer does not match the dose written on the drug chart, then re-check your calculation. If the answer is still the same, then inform the doctor and, if necessary, calculate the correct rate.

A formula can be derived:

$$mcg/kg/min = \frac{rate\,(mL/hour) \times amount\,of\,drug \times 1,000}{weight\,(kg) \times volume\,(mL) \times 60}$$

where in this case:

$$rate = 3.5\,mL/hour$$
$$amount\,of\,drug\,(mg) = 250\,mg$$
$$weight\,(kg) = 73\,kg$$
$$volume\,(mL) = 50\,mL$$
$$60\,converts\,minutes\,to\,hours$$
$$1,000\,converts\,mg\,to\,mcg$$

Substitute the numbers in the formula:

$$\frac{3.5 \times 250 \times 1,000}{73 \times 50 \times 60} = 3.99\,mcg/kg/min$$

This can be rounded up to 4 mcg/kg/min.

If the dose is given as a total dose and not on a weight basis, then the patient's weight is not needed:

$$mcg/min = \frac{rate\,(mL/hour) \times amount\,of\,drug \times 1,000}{volume\,(mL) \times 60}$$

Note: If the dose is in terms of milligrams, then there is no need to multiply by 1,000 (i.e. delete from the formula).

PROBLEMS

Convert each of the following infusion pump rates to a mcg/kg/min dose:

Question 14 You have dopamine 200 mg in 50 mL and the rate at which the pump is running is 4 mL/hour. The prescribed dose is 3 mcg/kg/min.

What dose is the pump delivering? (Patient's weight = 89 kg)

If the dose is wrong, at which rate should the pump be set?

Question 15 You have dobutamine 250 mg in 50 mL and the rate at which the pump is running is 5.4 mL/hour. The prescribed dose is 6 mcg/kg/min.

What dose is the pump delivering? (Patient's weight = 64 kg)

If the dose is wrong, at which rate should the pump be set?

Question 16 You have dopexamine 50 mg in 50 mL and the rate at which the pump is running is 28 mL/hour. The prescribed dose is 6 mcg/kg/min.

What dose is the pump delivering? (Patient's weight = 78 kg)

If the dose is wrong, at which rate should the pump be set?

Answers can be found on page 208.

CALCULATING THE LENGTH OF TIME FOR IV INFUSIONS

It may sometimes be necessary to calculate the number of hours an infusion should run at a specified rate. Also, it is a good way of checking your calculated drip rate or pump rate for an infusion.

For example: you are asked to give a litre of 5% glucose over 8 hours.

You have calculated that the drip rate should be 42 drops/min (using a standard giving set: 20 drops/mL) or 125 mL/hour for a pump.

To check your answer, you can calculate how long the infusion should take at the calculated rate. If your answers do not correspond (the answer should be 8 hours), then you have made an error and should re-check your calculation.

Alternatively, you can use this type of calculation to check the rate of an infusion already running.

For example: if an infusion is supposed to run over 6 hours, and the infusion is nearly finished after 4 hours, you can check the rate by calculating how long the infusion should take using that drip rate or the rate set on the pump. If the calculated answer is less than 6 hours, then the original rate was wrong and the doctor should be informed.

WORKED EXAMPLE

MANUALLY CONTROLLED INFUSIONS

The doctor prescribes 1 litre of 5% glucose to be given over 8 hours. The drip rate for the infusion is calculated to be 42 drops/min. You wish to check the drip rate; how many hours is the infusion going to run? (SGS = 20 drops/mL)

In this calculation, you first convert the volume being infused to drops; then calculate how long it will take at the specified rate.

STEP ONE

First, convert the volume to drops by multiplying the volume of the infusion (in mL) by the number of drops/mL for the giving set:

$$\text{volume of infusion} = 1 \text{ litre} = 1,000 \text{ mL}$$
$$1,000 \times 20 = 20,000 \text{ drops}$$

STEP TWO

From the rate, calculate how many minutes it will take for 1 drop:

$$42 \text{ drops per minute}$$
$$1 \text{ drop} = \frac{1}{42} \text{ min}$$

STEP THREE

Calculate how many minutes it will take to infuse the total number of drops:

$$1 \text{ drop} = \frac{1}{42} \text{ min}$$

$$20,000 \text{ drops} = \frac{1}{42} \times 20,000 = 476 \text{ min}$$

STEP FOUR

Convert minutes to hours by dividing by 60.

$$476 \text{ min} = \frac{476}{60} = 7.93 \text{ hours}$$

How much is 0.93 of an hour?

Multiply by 60 to convert part of an hour back to minutes:

$$0.93 \times 60 = 55.8 = 56 \text{ min (approx.)}$$

ANSWER: 1 litre of glucose 5% at a rate of 42 drops/min will take approximately 8 hours to run (7 hours and 56 minutes).

A formula can be used:

$$\text{number of hours the infusion is to run} =$$
$$\frac{\text{volume of the infusion}}{\text{rate (drops/min)} \times 60} \times \text{drip rate of giving set}$$

where in this case:

$$\text{volume of the infusion} = 1,000 \text{ mL}$$
$$\text{rate (drops/min)} = 42 \text{ drops/min}$$
$$\text{drip rate of giving set} = 20 \text{ drops/mL}$$
$$60 \text{ converts minutes to hours}$$

Substituting the numbers into the formula:

$$\frac{1,000}{42 \times 60} \times 20 = 7.94 \text{ hours}$$

Convert 0.94 hours to minutes: = 56 mins (approx.)

ANSWER: 1 litre of glucose 5% at a rate of 42 drops/min will take approximately 8 hours to run (7 hours 56 minutes).

WORKED EXAMPLE

INFUSION OR SYRINGE PUMPS

The doctor prescribes 1 litre of 5% glucose to be given over 8 hours. The rate for the infusion is calculated to be 125 mL/hour. You wish to check the rate; how many hours is the infusion going to run?

This is a simple calculation. You divide the total volume (in mL) by the rate to give the time over which the infusion is to run:

$$\text{calculated rate} = 125\,\text{mL/hour}$$
$$\text{volume} = 1,000\,\text{mL} \,(1\,\text{litre} = 1000\,\text{mL})$$
$$\frac{1,000}{125} = 8\,\text{hours}$$

ANSWER: 1 litre of glucose 5% at a rate of 125 mL/hour will take 8 hours to run.

A simple formula can be used:

$$\text{number of hours the infusion is to run} = \frac{\text{volume of the infusion}}{\text{rate (mL/hour)}}$$

where in this case:

$$\text{volume of the infusion} = 1,000\,\text{mL}$$
$$\text{rate (mL/hour)} = 125\,\text{mL/hour}$$

Substituting the numbers into the formula:

$$\frac{1,000}{125} = 8\,\text{hours}$$

ANSWER: 1 litre of glucose 5% at a rate of 125 mL/hour will take 8 hours to run.

PROBLEMS

Question 17 A 500 mL infusion of sodium chloride 0.9% is being given over 4 hours. The rate at which the infusion is being run is 42 drops/min.

How long will the infusion run at the specified rate (SGS)?

Question 18 A 1 litre infusion of sodium chloride 0.9% is being given over 12 hours. The rate at which the infusion is being run is 83 mL/hour.

How long will the infusion run at the specified rate?

Question 19 Isosorbide dinitrate is to be given at a dose of 2 mg/hour. At what rate should the pump be set (mL/hour) to give this dose using a 0.05%w/v solution?

Question 20 A patient is receiving flucloxacillin 1 g in 100 mL sodium chloride 0.9% four times a day. Each 500 mg vial of flucloxacillin contains 1.13 mmol sodium.

How many mmol of sodium is the patient receiving in 24 hours? (Sodium chloride 0.9% contains 154 mmol sodium per litre.)

Answers can be found on page 212.

OBJECTIVES
At the end of this chapter, you should be familiar with the following:
- Pharmacokinetics and pharmacodynamics
  - Absorption
  - Metabolism
  - Distribution
  - Elimination
- Administration of medicines
  - Oral
  - Parenteral
- NPSA guidelines promoting the safer use of injectable medicines

KEY POINTS

In order for a drug to reach its site of action and have an effect, it needs to enter the bloodstream. This is influenced by the route of administration and how the drug is absorbed.

Phamacokinetics and Pharmacodynamics

Pharmacokinetics examines the way in which the body 'handles drugs' and looks at:
- absorption of drugs into the body;
- distribution around the body;
- elimination or excretion.

Pharmacodynamics is the study of the mode of action of drugs – how they exert their effect.

Administration of Medicines

Which route of administration?
The route of administration depends upon:
- which is the most convenient route for the patient;
- the drug and its properties;
- the formulations available;
- how quick an effect is required;
- whether a local or systemic effect is required;
- the clinical condition of the patient – the oral route may not be possible;
- whether the patient is compliant or not.

Oral administration

For most patients, the oral route is the most convenient and acceptable method of taking medicines. Drugs may be given as tablets, capsules or liquids: other means include buccal or sublingual administration.

Parenteral administration of drugs

This is the injection of drugs directly into the blood or tissues. The three most common methods are: intravenous (IV), subcutaneous (SC) and intramuscular (IM).

Promoting the Safer Use of Injectable Medicines

The risks associated with using injectable medicines in clinical areas have been recognized and well known for some time. Recent research evidence indicates that the incidence of errors in prescribing, preparing and administering injectable medicines is higher than for other forms of medicine. As a consequence the National Patient Safety Agency (NPSA) issued safety alert 20: *Promoting Safer Use of Injectable Medicines* in March 2007. The alert covers multi-professional safer practice standards, with particular emphasis on prescribing, preparation and administration of injectable medicines in clinical areas.

- Take care when reading doses, either prescribed or found in the literature.
- Total daily dose (TDD) is the total dose and needs to be divided by the number of doses per day to give a single dose.
- To be sure that your answer is correct, it is best to calculate from first principles (for example, using the 'one unit rule').
- If using a formula, make sure that the figures are entered correctly.
- Ensure that everything is in the same units.
- Ask yourself whether your answer seems reasonable.
- **Always** re-check your answer – if in any doubt, **stop** and get help.

INTRODUCTION

The aim of this part of the book is to look at the administration of medicines with the emphasis on applying the principles learnt during the sections on drug calculations.

We will look at:

- pharmacokinetics and pharmacodynamics;
- common routes of administration;
- sources and interpretation of drug information.

In order for a drug to reach its site of action and have an effect, it needs to enter the bloodstream. This is influenced by the route of administration and how the drug is absorbed.

PHARMACOKINETICS AND PHARMACODYNAMICS

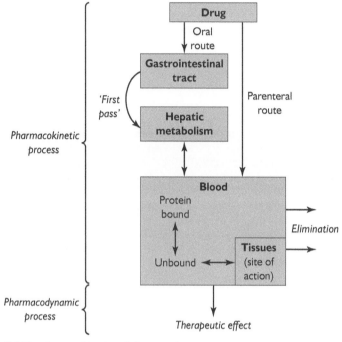

Fig 9.1 The pharmacokinetic and pharmacodynamic processes

Pharmacokinetics

The following is a brief introduction to a complex subject. The aim is to give you a general idea of the processes involved and to give an explanation of some of the terms used.

If a drug is going to have an effect in the body it needs to be present:

- in the right place;
- at the right concentration;
- for the right amount of time.

Pharmacokinetics examines the way in which the body 'handles drugs' and looks at:

- absorption of drugs into the body;
- distribution around the body;
- elimination or excretion.

It is an active (kinetic) process where all three processes occur at the same time. Knowing about the pharmacokinetics of a drug allows us to determine:

- what dose to give;
- how often to give it;
- how to change the dose in certain medical conditions;
- how some drug interactions occur.

Absorption

For a drug to be absorbed it needs to enter the systemic circulation. The oral route is the most commonly used and convenient method of administration for drugs. But some drugs are degraded by the acid content of the gastrointestinal (GI) tract and therefore cannot be given orally, e.g. insulin.

So how is a drug absorbed orally? Most drugs are absorbed by diffusion through the wall of the intestine into the bloodstream. In order to achieve this, the drug needs to pass through a cell membrane.

Drugs diffuse across cell membranes from a region of high concentration (GI tract) to one of low concentration (blood). The rate of diffusion depends not only on these differences in concentration, but also on the physiochemical properties of the drug. Cell membranes have a lipid or fatty layer, so drugs that can dissolve in this layer (lipid-soluble) can pass through easily. Drugs that are not lipid-soluble will not pass readily across the cell membrane. However, some drugs are transported across the cell membrane by carrier proteins (facilitated diffusion) or actively transported across by a pump system (active transport).

Other factors that affect absorption include the rate at which the GI tract empties (gastric motility or emptying time) and the presence or absence of food in the stomach. The speed of gastric emptying determines the speed at which the drug reaches its site of absorption.

Bioavailability

Bioavailability is a term that is used to describe the amount (sometimes referred to as the fraction) of the administered dose that reaches the systemic circulation of the patient. It is used generally in reference to drugs given by the oral route, although it can also refer to other routes of administration.

Thus, the bioavailability of a drug can be affected by:

- how the drug is absorbed;
- extent of drug metabolism before reaching systemic circulation – known as first-pass metabolism (see later);
- the drug's formulation and manufacture – this can affect the way a medicine disintegrates and dissolves;

- route of administration – drugs given by intravenous injection are said to have 100% bioavailability when compared to drugs given orally;
- other factors – age, sex, physical activity, genetic type, stress, malabsorption disorders, or previous GI surgery.

Metabolism

All drugs that are absorbed from the GI tract are transported to the liver, which is the main site for drug breakdown or metabolism, before reaching the general circulation and their site of action. Drugs can undergo several changes (first-pass metabolism). Some drugs:

- pass through the liver unchanged;
- are converted to an inactive form or metabolite which is excreted;
- are converted to an active form or metabolite which has an effect in its own right.

As a result of first-pass metabolism, only a fraction of drug may eventually reach the tissues to have a therapeutic effect.

If the drug is given parenterally, the liver is bypassed and so the amount of drug that reaches the circulation is greater than through oral administration. As a consequence, much smaller parenteral doses are needed to produce equivalent effect. For example, consider propranolol: if given IV, the standard dose is 1 mg; if given orally, the dose is 40 mg or higher.

Some metabolites of drugs are excreted into the biliary tract with bile and delivered back to the gut where they can be reactivated by gut bacteria; this reactivated drug can be reabsorbed and the cycle continues (enterohepatic circulation). The effect of this is to create a 'reservoir' of re-circulating drug and prolong its duration of action, e.g. morphine.

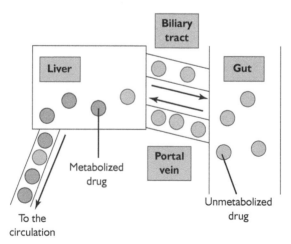

Fig 9.2 First-pass metabolism

Enzyme-inducing or -inhibiting drugs

Some drugs increase the production of enzymes in the liver (enzyme inducers, e.g. carbamazepine) that break down drugs – so a larger dose of affected drug is needed for a therapeutic effect. Other drugs may inhibit or reduce enzyme production (enzyme inhibitors, e.g. erythromycin) which reduces the rate at which another drugs are activated or inactivated – so a smaller dose of affected drug is needed for a therapeutic effect.

Distribution

After a drug enters the systemic circulation, it is distributed to the body's tissues. Movement from the circulation to the tissues is affected by a numbers of factors:

- rate of blood flow to the tissues;
- amount and/or type of tissue;
- the way in which blood and tissues interact with each other (partition characteristics);
- plasma proteins.

Plasma protein binding of drugs

The extent to which a drug is distributed into tissues depends on the extent of plasma protein and tissue binding. Once drugs are present in the bloodstream, they are transported partly in solution as free (unbound) drug and partly reversibly bound to plasma proteins (e.g. albumin, glycoproteins and lipoproteins).

When drugs are bound to plasma proteins they:

- do not undergo first-pass metabolism as only the unbound drug can be metabolized;
- have no effect because only free (unbound) fraction of the drug can enter into the tissues to exert an effect (the drug–protein complex is unable to cross cell membranes).

This drug–protein complex acts a reservoir as it can dissociate or separate and replace drug as it is removed or excreted. As a consequence, an equilibrium is set up between bound and unbound (free) drug. The degree of protein binding will thus determine the amount, time at, and thus efficacy at the target site.

In practice, changes in binding, resulting in increased levels of unbound drug, are important only for highly bound drugs with a narrow therapeutic index. The term *narrow therapeutic index* is used to describe drugs for which the toxic level is only slightly above the therapeutic range, and a slight increase in unbound drug may therefore result in adverse effects. An example is the anticoagulant warfarin, for which even a small change in binding will greatly affect the amount of free drug. Such an effect is produced by the concurrent administration of aspirin, which displaces warfarin and increases the amount of free anticoagulant.

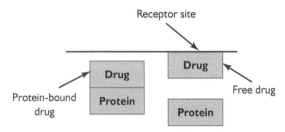

Fig 9.3 Protein binding

If a patient suffers from a condition in which plasma proteins are deficient (e.g. liver disease, malnutrition), more of the drug is free to enter the tissues. A normal dose of a drug could then be dangerous, because so little is bound by available protein, thus increasing the availability of unbound drug.

Volume of distribution
Drugs are distributed unevenly between various body fluids and tissues according to their physical and chemical properties. The term *volume of distribution* is used to reflect the amount of drug left in the bloodstream (plasma) after all the drug has been absorbed and distributed.

If a drug is 'held' in the bloodstream, it will have a small volume of distribution. If very little drug remains in the bloodstream, it has a large volume of distribution. We have to estimate values because we can only measure the drug concentration in the bloodstream and so it is known as the 'apparent' volume of distribution.

Elimination
There are various routes by which drugs can be eliminated from the body: the most important are the kidneys and the liver; while the least important are the biliary system, skin, lungs and gut. Primarily, drugs are eliminated from the body by a combination of renal excretion (main route) and hepatic metabolism.

Relative importance of metabolism and excretion in drug clearance
Depending upon their properties, some drugs mainly undergo metabolic clearance (liver) or renal clearance. Lipid-soluble drugs can readily cross cell membranes and are more likely to enter liver cells and undergo extensive hepatic clearance. However, if a drug is water-soluble, it will not be able to enter liver cells easily, so it is more likely to be eliminated by the kidneys. Only water-soluble drugs are eliminated by the kidneys; lipid-soluble drugs need to be metabolized to water-soluble metabolites before they can be excreted by the kidneys. If a lipid-soluble drug is filtered by the kidneys, it is largely reabsorbed in the tubules.

The excretion of drugs by the kidneys utilizes three processes that occur in the nephron of the kidney:

- glomerular filtration;
- passive tubular reabsorption; and
- active tubular secretion into the kidney tubule

Thus:

Total renal excretion = excretion by filtration + excretion by secretion − retention by reabsorption

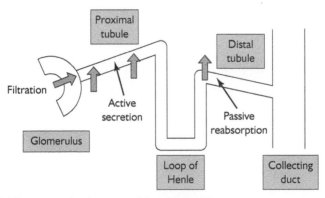

Fig 9.4 Excretion and reabsorption of drugs by the kidney

Drugs and/or their metabolized products are transported by the capillaries to the kidney tubule. Some drugs enter the tubule by glomerular filtration – this acts like a sieve allowing small drugs and those not bound to plasma protein to filter from the blood into the Bowman's capsule.

Most drugs enter the kidney tubule by means of active transport carriers.

Some drugs and their metabolites may be reabsorbed back into the bloodstream (this is referred to as passive diffusion since the process does not require energy). This occurs because water is reabsorbed back into the blood as a means of conserving body fluid. As this movement occurs, some drugs are transported along with it.

Half-life ($t_{1/2}$)

The duration of action of a drug is sometimes referred to its **half-life**. This is the period of time required for the concentration or amount of drug in the body to be reduced by one-half its original value. We usually consider the half-life of a drug in relation to the amount of the drug in plasma and this is influenced by the removal of a drug from the plasma (clearance) and the distribution of the drug in the various body tissues (volume of distribution).

Drugs that have short half-lives are cleared from the blood more rapidly than others, and so need to be given in regular doses to build up and maintain a high enough concentration in the blood to be therapeutically effective.

As repeated doses of a drug are administered, its plasma concentration builds up and reaches what is known as a **steady state**. This is when the concentration has reached a level that has a therapeutic effect and, as long as regular doses are given to counteract the amount being eliminated, it will continue to have an effect. The time taken to reach the steady state is about five times the half-life of a drug. Drugs such as digoxin and warfarin with a long half-life will take longer to reach a steady state than drugs with a shorter half-life.

Table 9.1 How the amount of drug in the body changes with half-life

NUMBER OF HALF-LIVES	AMOUNT OF DRUG CLEARED	AMOUNT OF DRUG IN THE BODY
1	50%	50%
2	25%	75%
3	12.5%	87.5%
4	6.25%	93.75%
5	3.125%	96.875%

You can see from Table 9.1 and Fig. 9.5 that after five half-lives, around 97 per cent of a single dose of a drug will be lost and 97 per cent of a drug will be present after repeated dosing.

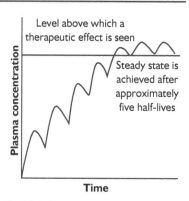

Fig 9.5 Achieving steady state

We can illustrate this by using a bucket to represent the body as a container and water to represent the drug. To be effective, the drug must reach a certain level and so must the water in the bucket, but the body is not a closed system – drug is constantly being lost. This loss of drug from the body can be represented by putting a small hole in the bucket so that some water is constantly leaking out. Like the drug level in the body, the level of water drops and needs to be topped up by giving regular doses.

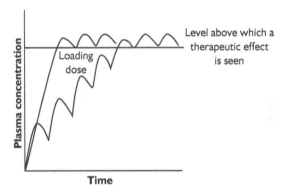

Fig 9.6 Effect of loading dose on steady state

Sometimes a **loading dose** may be administered so that a steady state is reached more quickly, then smaller 'maintenance' doses are given to ensure that the drug level stays within the steady state.

Pharmacodynamics

Pharmacodynamics is the study of the mode of action of drugs – how they exert their effect. There are receptors found on cell membranes or within a cell which natural hormones and neurotransmitters can bind to and cause a specific effect. Drugs can bind to these sites in ways that either cause an effect (agonists) or block an effect (antagonists). There is another way in which a drug may act: as partial agonists. A partial agonist does not produce a full effect – if there is a high concentration of partial agonists, they may bind to a receptor site without producing an effect. However, in doing so, they may block that receptor to other agonists and so act as an antagonist – so partial agonists have a 'dual' action.

Drugs can thus act by producing enhanced effects, e.g. salbutamol is a beta-2 receptor agonist that produces a bronchodilator effect in asthma by acting on the beta-2 receptors in smooth muscle cells.

Conversely, drugs can act by blocking a response, e.g. rantidine is an H_2 histamine receptor antagonist. One action of histamine is to stimulate gastric secretion. Ranitidine can block the action of histamine, reducing gastric acid secretion by about 70 per cent.

Another way in which drugs can act by interfering with cell processes is by affecting enzymes – enzymes can promote or accelerate biochemical reactions and the action of a drug depends upon the role of the enzyme it affects. For example, uric acid is produced by the enzyme xanthine oxidase, which is inhibited by allopurinol. High levels of uric acid can produce symptoms of gout and allopurinol works by reducing the synthesis of uric acid.

Drugs can affect transport processes – transport of certain substances, e.g. organic acids, cations (such as sodium, potassium and calcium) and neurotransmitters play an important role, and inhibition of their transport can have an effect. For example, thiazide diuretics reduce the reabsorption of sodium by the kidney tubules, resulting in an increased excretion of sodium and hence water.

Cancer drugs act by interfering with cell growth and division; antibiotics act by interfering with the cell processes of invading bacteria and other micro-organisms.

References

MH Beer, RS Porter and TV Jones. *The Merck Manual of Diagnosis and Therapy* (2006). Elsevier Health Sciences, Whitehouse Station, NJ, 18th ed.

G Downie, J Mackenzie and A Williams. *Pharmacology and Medicines Management for Nurses* (2008). Churchill Livingstone, Edinburgh, 4th ed.

B Greenstein and D Gould. *Trounce's Clinical Pharmacology for Nurses* (2004). Churchill Livingstone, Edinburgh, 17th ed.

SJ Hopkins. *Drugs and Pharmacology for Nurses* (1999). Churchill Livingstone, Edinburgh, 13th ed.

ME Winter. *Basic Clinical Pharmacokinetics* (2004). Lippincott Williams & Wilkins, Philadelphia, 4th ed.

ADMINISTRATION OF MEDICINES

There are several routes of administration, depending on:

- which is the most convenient route for the patient;
- the drug and its properties;
- the formulations available;
- how quick an effect is required;
- whether a local or systemic effect is required;
- clinical condition of the patient – the oral route may not be possible;
- whether the patient is compliant or not.

We will look at two of the most common routes of administration: oral and parenteral.

Oral administration

For most patients, the oral route is the most convenient and acceptable method of taking medicines. Drugs may be given as tablets, capsules or liquids; other means include buccal or sublingual administration.

The **advantages** of oral administration are that:

- it is convenient and allows self-administration;
- it is cheap as there is no need for special equipment;
- it avoids fear of needles;
- the GI tract provides a large surface area for absorption.

The **disadvantages** are that:

- absorption can be variable due to:
  - presence of food;
  - interactions;
  - gastric emptying;
- there is a risk of 'first-pass' metabolism;
- there is a need to remember to take doses.

As mentioned before, a major disadvantage of the oral route is that drugs can undergo 'first-pass' metabolism; taking medicines by the sublingual or buccal route avoids this as the medicines enter directly into the bloodstream through the oral mucosa.

With sublingual administration the drug is put under the tongue where it dissolves in salivary secretions; with buccal administration the drug is placed between the gum and the mucous membrane of the cheek. Absorption can be rapid, so drug effects can be seen within a few minutes, e.g. sublingual glyceryl trinitrate (GTN) tablets.

Practical implications

Liquid medicines are usually measured with a 5 mL spoon. For other doses, oral syringes or medicine measures are used.

1 Medicine measures – these are used on the ward to measure individual patient doses. They measure volumes ranging from 5 mL to 30 mL, and are not meant to be accurate. The graduation mark to which you are measuring should be at eye level. If viewed from above, the level may appear higher than it really is; if viewed from below, it appears lower.
2 Oral syringes – these are useful for measuring doses less than 5 mL. Oral syringes are available in various sizes, an example are the Baxa Exacta-Med® range.

Oral syringe calibrations

You should use the most appropriate syringe for your dose, and calculate doses according to the syringe graduations. For example:

SYRINGE SIZE	GRADUATIONS	CALCULATE DOSE (mL)
0.5 mL, 1 mL	0.01 mL	**Two** decimal places
2 mL, 3 mL	0.1 mL	**One** decimal place
5 mL, 10 mL	0.2 mL	Round up or down to the nearest multiple of 0.2 mL
20 mL, 35 mL, 60 mL	1 mL	Round up or down to the nearest mL

As with syringes for parenteral use, you should not try to administer the small amount of liquid that is left in the nozzle of the syringe after administering the drug. This small volume is known as 'dead space' or 'dead volume'. However, there are concerns with this 'dead space' when administering small doses and to babies; the 'dead space' has a greater volume that that for syringes meant for parenteral use. If a baby is allowed to suck on an oral syringe, then there is a danger that the baby will suck all the medicine out of the syringe (including the amount contained in the 'dead space') and may inadvertently take too much.

A part of the oral syringe design is that it should not be possible to attach a needle to the nozzle of the syringe. This prevents the accidental intravenous administration of an oral preparation. The problem was highlighted by the National Patient Safety Agency (NPSA) bulletin: *Promoting Safer Measurement and Administration of Liquid Medicines via Oral and Other Enteral Routes* (March 2007) – available on-line at: http://www.npsa.nhs.uk/nrls/alerts-and-directives/alerts/liquid-medicines/

Parenteral administration of drugs

Parenteral administration is the injection of drugs directly into the blood or tissues. The three most common methods are: intravenous (IV), subcutaneous (SC) and intramuscular (IM).

Intravenous (IV) injection

The drug is injected directly into a vein, usually in the arm or hand.

Administering drugs by the IV route can be associated with problems; so a definite decision must be made to use the IV route and it should only be used if no other route is appropriate. Situations in which IV therapy would be appropriate are when:

- the patient is unable to take or tolerate oral medication, or has problems with absorption;
- high drug levels are needed rapidly which cannot be achieved by another route because they:
  - are not absorbed orally;
  - are inactivated by the gut;
  - or undergo extensive first-pass-metabolism.
- constant drug levels are needed (such as those achieved by a continuous infusion);

- drugs have a very short elimination half-life ($t_{1/2}$). Remember, from the section on pharmacokinetics, the elimination half-life is the time taken for the concentration or level of a drug in the blood or plasma to fall to half its original value. Drugs with very short half-lives disappear from the bloodstream very quickly and may need to be administered by a continuous infusion to maintain a clinical effect.

The **advantages** of IV injection are that:

- a rapid onset of action and response is achieved since it bypasses the GI tract and first-pass metabolism;
- a constant and predictable therapeutic effect can be attained;
- it can be used for drugs that are irritant or unpredictable when administered IM (e.g. patients with small muscle mass, who may have thrombocytopenia, or have haemophilia);
- it allows administration when the oral route cannot be used (e.g. when patients are nil-by-mouth, at risk of aspiration or suffering from nausea and vomiting);
- it enables drugs to be administered to patients who are unconscious;
- it quickly corrects fluid and electrolyte imbalances.

The **disadvantages** are that:

- training is required – not only on how to use the equipment, but also on how to for calculate doses and rates of infusion;
- several risks are associated with the IV route:
  - toxicity – side effects usually more immediate and severe;
  - accidental overdose;
  - embolism;
  - microbial contamination/infection;
  - phlebitis/thrombophlebitis;
  - extravasation;
  - particulate contamination;
  - fluid overload;
  - compatibility/stability problems.

Methods of intravenous administration

Intravenous bolus

This is the administration of a small volume (usually up to 10 mL) into a cannula or the injection site of an administration set – over 3–5 minutes unless otherwise specified.

Indications for use of an IV bolus are:

- to achieve immediate and high drug levels – as needed in an emergency;
- to ensure that medicines that are inactivated very rapidly, e.g. adenosine used to treat arrthymias, produce a clinical effect.

Drawbacks to use are:

- only small volumes can be administered;
- the dose may be administered too rapidly, which may be associated with increased adverse events for some medicines, e.g. vancomycin ('red man syndrome');
- the administration is unlikely to be able to be stopped if an adverse event occurs;
- damage to the veins, e.g. phlebitis or extravasation, especially with potentially irritant medicines.

Intermittent intravenous infusion

This is the administration of a small volume infusion (usually up to 250 mL) over a given time (usually 20 minutes to 2 hours), either as a one-off dose or repeated at specific time intervals. It is often a compromise between a bolus injection and continuous infusion in that it can achieve high plasma concentrations rapidly to ensure clinical efficacy and yet reduce the risk of adverse reactions associated with rapid administration.

Continuous intravenous infusion

This is the administration of a larger volume (usually between 500 mL and 3 litres) over a number of hours. Continuous infusions are usually used to replace fluids and to correct electrolyte imbalances. Sometimes, drugs are added in order to produce a constant effect, e.g. as with analgesics – usually given as small-volume infusions (e.g. 50 mL) via syringe drivers.

Indications for use of *intermittent* infusions are:

- when a drug must be diluted in a volume of fluid larger than is practical for a bolus injection;
- when plasma levels need to be higher than those that can be achieved by continuous infusion;
- when a faster response is required than can be achieved by a continuous infusion;
- when a drug would be unstable when given as a continuous infusion.

Indications for use of *continuous* infusions are:

- when a constant therapeutic effect is required or to maintain adequate plasma concentrations;
- when a medicine has a rapid elimination rate or short half-life and therefore can have an effect only if given continuously.

Drawbacks to use of intermittent or continuous infusions are:

- volume of diluent may cause fluid overload in susceptible patients, e.g. the elderly, those with heart or renal failure;

- incompatibility problems with the infusion fluid;
- incomplete mixing of solutions;
- training is required – calculation skills for accurate determination of infusion concentration and rates; knowledge of, and competence in, operating infusion devices;
- increased risk of microbial and particulate contamination during preparation;
- risk of complications, such as haematoma, phlebitis and extravasation.

Subcutaneous (SC) injection

The SC route is generally used for administering small volumes (up to 2 mL) of non-irritant drugs such as insulin or heparin. Subcutaneous injections are usually given into the fatty layer directly below the skin; absorption is greater when compared with the oral route as the drug will be absorbed via the capillaries.

The **advantages** of SC injection are that:

- the patient can self-administer;
- first-pass metabolism is avoided.

The **disadvantages** are that:

- care must be taken not to inject IV;
- complications can arise, e.g. bruising.

Intramuscular (IM) injection

The IM route is generally used for the administration of drugs in the form of suspensions or oily solutions (usually no more than 3 mL). Absorption from IM injections can be variable and depends upon which muscle is used and the rate of perfusion through the muscle (this can be increased by gently massaging the site of the injection).

The **advantages** of IM injection are that:

- it is easier to give than an IV infusion;
- first-pass metabolism is avoided;
- a depot effect is possible.

The **disadvantages** are that:

- injection can be painful;
- self-administration is difficult;
- complications can arise, e.g. bruising or abscesses.

Practical aspects

As with oral syringes, syringes for parenteral use are available in various sizes. Once again, you should use the most appropriate syringe for your dose, and calculate doses according to the syringe. For example:

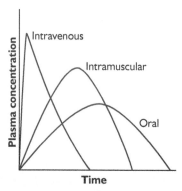

Fig 9.7 Plasma profiles of drugs administered via different routes

SYRINGE SIZE	GRADUATIONS	CALCULATE DOSE (mL)
1 mL	0.01 mL	**Two** decimal places
2 mL	0.1 mL	**One** decimal place
5 mL	0.2 mL	Round up or down to the nearest multiple of 0.2 mL
10 mL	0.5 mL	Round up or down to the nearest multiple of 0.5 mL
20 mL, 30 mL, 50 mL	1 mL	Round up or down to the nearest mL

As with syringes for oral use, there is also a 'dead space' or 'dead volume' with an associated volume which is taken into account by the manufacturer. When measuring a volume with a syringe, it is important to expel all the air first before adjusting to the final volume. The volume is measured from the bottom of the plunger.

You should not try to administer the small amount of liquid that is left in the nozzle of the syringe after administering the drug – 'dead space' or 'dead volume'. However, there are concerns with this 'dead space' when administering small doses and to babies, particularly if the dose is diluted before administration. For example: if a drug is drawn up to the 0.02 mL mark of a 1 mL syringe and injected directly, the drug in the dead space is retained in the syringe, and there is no overdose delivered. However, when a diluent is drawn up into the syringe for dilution, the drug in the dead space is also drawn up, and this results in possible overdosing.

PROMOTING THE SAFER USE OF INJECTABLE MEDICINES

The risks associated with using injectable medicines in clinical areas have been recognized and well known for some time. Evidence indicates that the incidence of errors in prescribing, preparing and administering injectable medicines is higher than for other forms of medicine. As a consequence the National Patient Safety Agency (NPSA) issued safety alert 20: *Promoting Safer Use of Injectable Medicines* in March 2007. The alert covers multi-professional safer practice standards, with particular emphasis on prescribing, preparation and administration of injectable medicines in clinical areas.

The NPSA has produced a risk assessment tool which highlights eight risks associated with the prescribing, preparation and administration of injectable drugs.

There are two risks that highlight the involvement of calculations and so emphasize the need to be able to perform calculations confidently and competently; these risks are:

- **Complex calculations**: any calculation with more than one step required for preparation and/or administration, e.g. microgram/kg/hour, dose unit conversion such as mg to mmol or % to mg.
- **Use of a pump or syringe driver**: all pumps and syringe drivers require some element of calculation and therefore have potential for error and should be included in the risk factors. However, it is important to note that this potential risk is considered less significant than the risks associated with not using a pump when indicated.

Each injectable drug in use within a particular hospital needs to undergo a risk assessment using a set proforma. Once risks have been identified, action plans need to be developed to minimize them.

Hospitals must ensure that healthcare staff who prescribe, prepare and administer injectable medicines have received training and have the necessary work competences to undertake their duties safely. This will include IV study days which will teach and assess nurses so that they are able to prepare and administer injectable drugs – part of these assessments will involve drug calculations.

References

http://www.npsa.nhs.uk/nrls/alerts-and-directives/alerts/injectable-medicines/
Injectable Administration of Medicines (2007). Pharmacy Department, UCL Hospitals. Blackwell Publishing: Oxford, 2nd ed.

Injectable drug risk assessment proforma

Risk assessment summary for high- and moderate-risk injectable medicines products			Directorate:										Date:	
Risk factors														
Prepared injectable medicine	Strength	Diluent	Final volume	Bag/syringe	Therapeutic	Use of concentrate	Complex calculation	Complex preparation	Reconstitute vial	Part/multiple container	Infusions pump or driver	Non-standard infusion set	Risk assessment score	Risk reduction method(s)	Revised score
					✓	✓	✓	✓	✓	✓	✓	✓			
Risk assessment undertaken by:			Name of pharmacist:					Name of clinical practioner:							

PROBLEMS

Write down the volume as indicated on the following syringes for oral use:

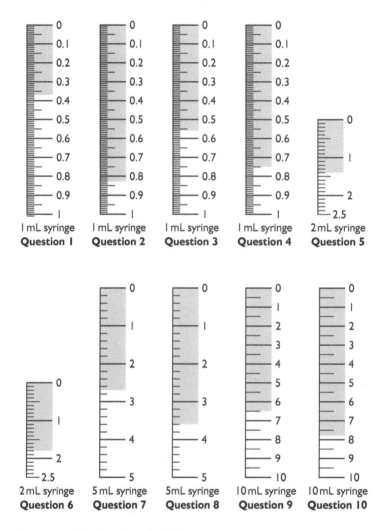

Answers can be found on page 215.

OBJECTIVES

At the end of this chapter, you should be familiar with the following:

- Gravity devices
- Pumped systems
  - Volumetric pumps
  - Syringe pumps
  - Patient-controlled analgesia (PCA)
  - Anaesthesia pumps
  - Pumps for ambulatory use
- Infusion device classification

KEY POINTS

Various devices are available.

Gravity Devices

- These depend entirely on gravity to drive the infusion; flow is measured by counting the drops.
- A gravity device should be considered only for low-risk infusions such as sodium chloride, dextrose saline and dextrose infusions.
- A gravity device should not be used for infusions:
  - containing potassium;
  - containing drug therapies requiring accurate monitoring or delivery of accurate volumes;
  - delivered to volume-sensitive patients.

Pumped Systems

These include the following different types:

Volumetric pumps

- Preferred pumps for medium and large flow rate and volume infusions; although some are designed specially to operate at low flow rates for neonatal use (not recommended for <5 mL/hour).

Syringe pumps

- These are used to administer drugs or infusions in small or medium volumes, and are calibrated at rates of 0.1 to 99 mL/hour (recommended for <5 mL/hour).
- Syringe pumps are used extensively where small volumes of highly concentrated drugs are required at low flow rates: usually in intensive care settings.

Patient-controlled analgesia (PCA) pumps

- These pumps are specifically designed for this purpose and are programmable to tailor analgesia for individual needs.

Anaesthesia pumps

- These are syringe pumps designed for use in anaesthesia or sedation and must be used *only* for this purpose; they are unsuitable for any other use. They should be restricted to operating and high dependency areas.

Pumps for ambulatory use

- Ambulatory pumps can be carried around by patients both in hospital and at home.

INTRODUCTION

This chapter is not meant to be an exhaustive review, but is a brief overview of the different infusion devices available and their use in drug administration. The reader is advised to seek more detailed references and to read the manufacturers' manuals for advice on setting up and using infusion devices, and problems associated with them.

In general, infusion pumps are capable of accurate delivery of solutions over a wide range of volumes and flow rates, and may be designed for specialist applications, e.g. for neonatal use.

GRAVITY DEVICES

Gravity devices depend entirely on gravity to drive the infusion; the pressure for the infusion depends on the height of the liquid above the infusion site. Flow is measured by counting the drops.

A gravity device should only be considered for low-risk infusions such as sodium chloride, dextrose saline and dextrose infusions. A gravity device should **not** be used for infusions containing potassium, or drug therapies requiring accurate monitoring or delivery of accurate volumes. Infusions, even low risk, should not be delivered to volume-sensitive patients via a gravity line but must be given via an infusion pump.

PUMPED SYSTEMS

Volumetric pumps

Volumetric pumps are the preferred pumps for medium and large flow rate and large volume infusions; although some are designed specially to operate at low flow rates for neonatal use. The rate is given in millilitres per hour (typical range 1–999 mL/hour).

Typically, most volumetric pumps will perform satisfactorily at rates down to 5 mL/hour. A syringe pump should be used for rates lower than 5 mL/hour or when short-term accuracy is required.

All volumetric pumps are designed to use a specific giving set. Using any set other than the correct one will result in reduced accuracy and poor alarm responses.

For delivery of low-risk infusions a gravity device should be considered rather than a volumetric pump, unless accurate monitoring is required, or the patient is at risk of fluid overload.

Syringe pumps

Syringe pumps are used to administer drugs or infusions in small or medium volumes, and are calibrated for delivery in millilitres per hour, typically 0.1 to 99 mL/hour. Syringe pumps have better short-term accuracy than volumetric pumps and are therefore typically superior when delivering drugs at rates below 5 mL/hour. Syringe pumps are used extensively where small volumes of highly concentrated drugs are required at low flow rates – usually in intensive care settings.

Patient-controlled analgesia (PCA) pumps

Patient-controlled analgesia (PCA) pumps are specifically designed to deliver analgesia to meet individual needs and to allow patients to have some control over their own analgesia. They are typically syringe pumps and the difference between a PCA pump and a normal syringe pump is that patients are able to deliver a bolus dose themselves. Clinical staff may program a PCA pump to deliver a pre-set bolus on demand, or have a pre-set lockout time between boluses. In addition, PCA pumps may also be programmed to deliver a basal (continuous, low rate) infusion.

Once programmed, access to the control of the pump is usually restricted. A feature of most PCA pumps is a memory log, which enables the clinician to determine when, and how often, the patient has made a demand and what total volume of drug has been infused over a given time.

Anaesthesia pumps

Anaesthesia pumps are syringe pumps designed for use in anaesthesia or sedation and must be used *only* for this purpose; they are unsuitable for any other use. They should be restricted to operating and high dependency areas.

Pumps for ambulatory use

Pumps for ambulatory use are miniature versions of syringe pumps which are battery driven. They deliver their dose in bursts, not in an even flow rate, almost like a continual sequence of micro-boluses.

Ambulatory pumps can be carried around by patients whether they are in hospital or at home.

The most common type is a syringe driver. They are typically used for pain control, cytotoxic therapy, heparin and insulin.

Syringe drivers

These pumps are designed to deliver drugs accurately over a certain period of time (usually 24 hours). They have the advantage of being small and compact, and so can be carried easily by the patient, avoiding the need for numerous injections throughout the day.

Various devices suitable for continuous subcutaneous infusion are available. It is not possible to give details of them all here. Most are battery operated but may differ in their method of operation, particularly for setting the delivery rate.

The SIMS Graseby syringe drivers type MS16A (blue panel) and type MS26 (green panel) are described here because they are widely used. This does not imply that these two models are any better than the others. It should be noted that syringe drivers are undergoing continual development and improvement.

There are two types of Graseby syringe drivers:

- MS16A (blue panel) – designed to deliver drugs at an hourly rate;
- MS26 (green panel) – designed to deliver drugs at a daily rate (i.e. over 24 hours).

To avoid confusion between the two pumps, the MS16A is clearly marked with a pink '1HR' in the bottom right-hand corner; the MS26 has an orange/brown '24HR' instead. Rate is set in terms of millimetres per hour or millimetres per day, that is, linear travel of syringe plunger against time.

Calculation of dose

The amount required is the total dose to be given over 24 hours.

- If the dose is prescribed in 'mg/hour', then it is necessary to calculate the total amount for 24 hours by multiplying by 24, e.g. if the dose is 3 mg/hour, then:

  total amount required for 24 hours = 3 × 24 = 72 mg

- If the dose is prescribed every 4 hours (or whatever), multiply the dose by the number of times the dose is given in 24 hours, i.e. if the dose is 20 mg every 4 hours:

  dose is being given 6 times in 24 hours

  (divide 24 by the dosing frequency, i.e. $\frac{24}{4} = 6$)

  total amount required for 24 hours = 20 × 6 = 120 mg

- If the dose is prescribed in 'mg/day' (24 hours), then no calculation is necessary, i.e. if the dose is 60 mg/day (24 hours), then:

$$\text{total amount required for 24 hours} = 60\,\text{mg}$$

To set the rate

Always set up a syringe driver to make the fluid length (*L* in Fig. 10.1) about 50 mm with diluent before priming the infusion set. Priming will take about 2 mm of this total, leaving 48 mm of fluid to be transfused over 24 hours. This makes the arithmetic of setting easier. When infusions do not require a priming volume, *L* should be set at 48 mm. The volume varies from one brand of syringe to another, but the dose and the distance *L* are the important factors, not the volume.

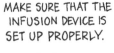

MAKE SURE THAT THE INFUSION DEVICE IS SET UP PROPERLY.

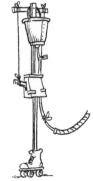

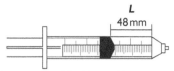

L

48 mm

Fig 10.1 Measurement of fluid length (*L*) in syringe

MS16A (blue panel) – mm/hour

$$\text{set rate} = \frac{\text{distance } L \text{ in mm (48)}}{\text{infusion time in hours}}$$

For example:

$$\frac{48\,\text{mm}}{24\,\text{hour}} = 2\,\text{mm/hour}$$

So the dial should read 02 mm/hour.

MS26 (green panel) – mm/24 hours

$$\text{set rate} = \frac{\text{distance } L \text{ in mm (48)}}{\text{infusion time in days}}$$

For example:

$$\frac{48\,\text{mm}}{1\,\text{day}} = 48\,\text{mm/day (24 hours)}$$

So the dial should read 48 mm/24 hours.

INFUSION DEVICE CLASSIFICATION

The Medicines and Healthcare Products Regulatory Agency (MHRA), formerly the Medical Devices Agency, has made recommendations on the safety and performance of infusion devices in order to enable users to make the appropriate choice of equipment to suit most applications. The new classification system is divided into three major categories according to the potential risks involved. A pump suited to the high-risk category of therapy (A) can be safely used for the other categories (B and C). A pump suited to category B can be used for B and C therapies, whereas a pump with the lowest specification (C) is suited only to category C therapies.

Hospitals will be required to label each infusion pump with its category and it will be necessary to know the category of the proposed therapy and match it with a pump of the same or better category.

THERAPY CATEGORY	THERAPY DESCRIPTION	PATIENT GROUP	CRITICAL PERFORMANCE PARAMETERS
A	Drugs with narrow therapeutic margin	Any	Good long-term accuracy Good short-term accuracy Rapid alarm after occlusion Small occlusion bolus Able to detect very small air embolus (volumetric pumps only) Small flow rate increments Good bolus accuracy Rapid start-up time (syringe pumps only)
	Drugs with short half-life	Any	
	Any infusion given to neonates	Neonates	
B	Drugs, other than those with a short half-life	Any, except neonates	Good long-term accuracy Alarm after occlusion Small occlusion bolus Able to detect small air embolus (volumetric pumps only) Small flow rate increments Bolus accuracy
	Total parenteral nutrition (TPN) Fluid maintenance Transfusions	Volume-sensitive, except neonates	
	Diamorphine	Any, except neonates	
C	TPN Fluid maintenance Transfusions	Any, except volume-sensitive or neonates	Long-term accuracy Alarm after occlusion Small occlusion bolus Able to detect air embolus (volumetric pumps only) Incremental flow rates

Errors involving the incorrect setting of IV pumps are amongst the most common errors reported. These errors involve volumetric infusion pumps as well as syringe driver and PCA pumps. Owing to the wide variety of uses for these devices, errors in setting the correct drug administration rates may involve narcotic analgesics, insulin, heparin, cardiovascular drugs and cancer chemotherapy agents. Although a fault with the equipment is frequently cited, testing the pumps after an error has occurred rarely shows that they are in fact faulty. In the vast majority of cases the fault is due to operator error.

It is important that calculations involving dosing and setting infusion rates are checked before using any infusion device.

OBJECTIVES

At the end of this chapter, you should be familiar with the following:

- Drug handling in children
- Routes of administration of drugs
    - Oral administration
    - Parenteral administration
- Practical implications
    - General
    - Dosing
    - Licensing and 'off-label' use
    - Formulations
    - Problems associated with paediatric doses
- Useful reference books
- Approximate values useful in the calculation of doses in children
- Calculating dosages

KEY POINTS

Prescribing in Paediatrics

- Doses are usually prescribed on a weight (mg/kg) or surface area (mg/m^2) basis; the use of formulae is no longer recommended.

Drug Handling and Drug Response

- Drug handling (pharmacokinetcs) and drug response (pharmacodynamics) may change, particularly in neonates.
- Standard (adult) doses of some drugs may have to be increased or reduced depending on how they are absorbed, broken down or metabolized, distributed or excreted.

Routes of Administration

- These are largely determined by the age of the child and how ill the child is.
    - In the sick premature newborn, almost all drugs are given IV.
    - In full-term newborns, and older children, the oral route is the easiest and most convenient route, particularly for long-term treatment. However, for the acutely ill child and for children with vomiting, diarrhoea and impaired gastrointestinal function, the parenteral route is recommended.

Practical Implications

- If possible, children should know why they need a medicine and be shown how they can take it.
- Young children and infants who cannot understand will usually take medicine from someone they know and trust – a parent or main carer.

> Therefore it is important that those who give medicines know about the medicine and how to give it.
> • Occasionally, there may be problems in giving medicines – usually due to taste, difficulty swallowing a tablet or capsule, or strengths of medicines available. In these cases a liquid preparation is necessary – either available commercially or specially made.
> • Some medicines, particularly commercially available ones, may contain excipients (e.g. alcohol) which may cause problems in children – prescribers and those administering medicines should take this into account.

INTRODUCTION

Children are very different from adults and shouldn't be considered as small adults when assessing the effect a medicine may have. This is certainly true for the way in which children handle and respond to drugs. An understanding of the likely changes that can occur as children grow is important for the administration of medicines – but also for an awareness of when children are able to swallow tablets, open bottles, read information and so on.

As knowledge has increased, the use of formulae to estimate children's doses based on those of adults is no longer recommended. Doses are given in terms of either body weight (mg/kg) or body surface area (mg/m²) in an attempt to take account of such developmental changes.

The International Committee on Harmonization (2000) has suggested that childhood be divided into the following age ranges for the purposes of clinical trials and licensing of medicines (see Table 11.1). These age ranges are intended to reflect biological changes.

Table 11.1 Age ranges and definitions

DEFINITION	AGE RANGE
Pre-term newborn infants	<37 weeks' gestation
Term newborn infants	0–27 days
Infants and toddlers	28 days to 23 months
Children	2–11 years
Adolescents	12–16 or 18 years

DRUG HANDLING IN CHILDREN

As stated earlier, children are different from adults in the way that they handle and respond to drugs. Age-related differences in drug handling (pharmacokinetics) and drug sensitivity (pharmacodynamics) occur throughout childhood and account for many of the differences between drug doses at various stages of childhood. Many drugs used in paediatrics have not been studied adequately or at all in children, so prescribing for children may not always be easy.

Drug absorption

There are various differences between children and adults that can affect the way in which drugs are absorbed orally. Changes in the gastric pH, which can affect the absorption of certain drugs, occur. In neonates, there is reduced gastric acid secretion and this means that the rate of absorption of acidic drugs may be decreased during this period and for non-acidic or basic drugs, the rate is expected to be increased. Otherwise, oral absorption in older infants (from 2 years) and children is similar to that in adults.

Another difference is a variation in the time taken for gastric emptying or for gastrointestinal (GI) transit – that is, the time taken for something to travel through the GI tract. There is also some evidence to suggest that in neonates and young infants, up to the age of 4–6 months, this may be prolonged (relative to adults and older children); resulting in slower rates of absorption and more time to achieve maximum plasma levels.

Vomiting or acute diarrhoea, which is particularly common during childhood, may dramatically reduce the extent of drug absorption, by reducing the time that the drug remains in the small intestine. This means that drugs may have a reduced effect and therefore may have to be given by another route.

Other factors affecting absorption include the immature biliary system, which may affect the absorption and transport of fat-soluble (lipophilic) drugs. In addition, the activity of drug-metabolizing enzymes in the liver and bacterial microflora in the gut may vary with age and this may lead to different and unpredictable oral drug absorption in neonates and young infants.

Drug distribution

The distribution of a drug to its site of action influences its therapeutic and adverse effects. This may vary considerably in neonates and young infants, resulting in a different therapeutic or adverse effect from that which is expected.

In general, changes in body composition (body water and fat) can alter the way that drugs are distributed round the body. The most dramatic changes occur in the first year of life but continue throughout puberty and adolescence, particularly the proportion of total body fat. The extent to which a drug distributes between fat and water depends upon its physicochemical properties, i.e. according to how it dissolves in water (water solubility) and in fat (lipid solubility). Water-soluble drugs are mainly distributed within the extracellular space and fat soluble drugs within fat.

Table 11.2 Relative amounts of body water and fat (as percentage of total body weight) at different ages

	PRE-TERM	FULL-TERM	INFANT (6 MONTHS)	CHILD	YOUNG ADULT	ELDERLY ADULT
Extracellular fluid	50%	40%	35%	25%	15%	10%
Total body water	85%	70%	70%	65%	60%	45%
Fat content	1%	15%	15%	15%	20%	10%

Neonates and infants have relatively large extracellular fluid and total body water spaces compared with adults. This results in a larger apparent volume of distribution of drugs that distribute into these spaces and lower plasma concentrations for the same weight-based dose, and so higher doses of water-soluble drugs are required.

Another major determinant of drug distribution is protein binding. A certain proportion of drug will be bound to plasma proteins and a proportion will be unbound – only the unbound drug is able to go to its site of action.

Protein binding is reduced in neonates, owing to reduced albumin and plasma protein concentrations, but increases with age and reaches adult levels by about one year.

For drugs that are highly protein bound, small changes in the binding of the drug can make a large difference to the free drug concentration if the drug is displaced. As a consequence, lower total plasma concentrations of some drugs may be required to achieve a therapeutic effect. Drugs affected include phenytoin, phenobarbital and furosemide.

This change in binding is also important with regards to bilirubin in neonates. Bilirubin is a breakdown product of old blood cells which is carried in the blood (by binding to plasma proteins) to the liver where it is chemically modified (by conjugation) and then excreted in the bile into the newborn's digestive tract. Displacement by drugs and the immature conjugating mechanisms of the liver means that unconjugated bilirubin levels can rise and can cross the brain–blood barrier; high levels cause kernicterus (brain damage). Conversely, high circulating bilirubin levels in neonates may displace drugs from proteins.

Metabolism

The primary organ for drug breakdown or metabolism is the liver. In the first weeks of life, the ability of the liver to metabolize drugs is not fully developed. This all changes in the 1–9-month age group in which the metabolic clearance of drugs is shown to be greater than in adults. This is probably due to the relatively large size of the liver compared with body size and maturation of the enzyme systems. Thus to achieve plasma concentrations similar to those seen in adults, dosing in this group may need to be higher.

Elimination

In neonates, the immaturity of the kidneys, particularly glomerular filtration and active tubular secretion and reabsorption of drugs, limits the ability to excrete drugs renally. Below 3–6 months of age, glomerular filtration is less than that of adults, but this may be partially compensated by a relatively greater reduction in tubular reabsorption as tubular function matures at a slower rate. However, drugs may accumulate, leading to toxic effects. Maturity of renal function occurs towards 6–8 months of age. After 8–12 months, renal function is similar to that seen in older children and adults.

ROUTES OF ADMINISTRATION OF DRUGS

These are largely determined mainly by the age of the child and how ill the child is. In the sick premature newborn, almost all drugs are given IV since GI function and therefore drug absorption are impaired. (Intramuscular, IM, administration is not suitable as there is very poor muscle mass.)

In full-term newborns, and older children, the oral route is the easiest and most convenient route, particularly for long-term treatment. However, for the acutely ill child and for children with vomiting, diarrhoea and impaired GI function, the parenteral route is recommended.

Oral administration

It is not always possible to give tablets or capsules: either the dose required does not exist, or the child cannot swallow tablets or capsules (children under 5 years are unlikely to accept tablets or capsules). Therefore an oral liquid preparation is necessary, either as a ready-made preparation, or one made especially by the pharmacy. Older children also often prefer liquids. Liquid formulations sometimes have the disadvantage of an unpleasant taste which may be disguised by flavouring or by mixing them with, or following them immediately by, favourite foods or drinks. However, mixing the drugs with food may cause dosage problems and affect absorption. It is worth remembering that, to ensure adequate dosing, all of the medicine and food must be taken.

Parents and carers should be discouraged from adding medicines to a baby's bottle. This is because of potential interactions with milk feeds and under dosing if not all the feed is taken. The crushing or opening of slow-release tablets and capsules should also be discouraged; it should only be done on advice from pharmacy.

Domestic teaspoons vary in size and are not a reliable measure. A 5 mL medicine spoon or oral syringe should be used and parents or carers may need to be shown how to use these (see the section on oral syringes in Chapter 9 'Action and administration of medicines', page 131).

Parenteral administration

The parenteral route is the most reliable with regards to obtaining predictable blood levels; giving drugs intravenously is the most commonly used parenteral route. It is now commonplace to use infusion pumps when giving infusions, as opposed to using a paediatric or micro-drop giving set on its own, as pumps are considered to be more accurate and safer.

Intramuscular (IM)

Most drugs can be injected into muscle, but the IM route should be avoided if at all possible owing to the pain it causes, and reduced muscle mass and poor muscle perfusion of blood in children. In practice the route is used for concentrated and irritating solutions that may cause local pain if injected subcutaneously and which cannot be given by any other way.

In a child who has already received several days of intravenous antibiotics and in whom cannulation has become difficult, two or three days of a once-daily IM injection to complete the course may be preferable to multiple intravenous cannulation attempts which may cause stress and distress to the child. Thin infants may be given 1–2 mL and bigger children 1–5 mL, using needles of appropriate length for the site chosen. The shorter and the narrower the needle, the less pain it will cause.

Intravenous (IV)

In hospital practice, drugs not given orally are usually given IV rather than SC or IM, as the effect is quicker and more predictable, the pain of multiple injections is avoided and larger volumes can be given. However, in neonates, owing to the fragility of the veins, extravasation is relatively common and can cause problems if drugs leak into the tissues. Central venous access is used for children who need irritant or cardiac drugs, administration of medicines over long periods and for home therapy with IV drugs.

PRACTICAL IMPLICATIONS

General

In the UK, the *British National Formulary for Children* (BNF-C) (see References below) is a national formulary that includes prescribing guidelines and drug monographs. You should read the relevant sections.

If possible, children should know why they need a medicine and be shown how they can take it. Young children and infants who cannot understand will usually take medicine from someone they know and trust – a parent or main carer. So it is important that those who give medicines know about the medicine and how to give it. Occasionally, there may be problems in giving medicines – usually due to taste or difficulty swallowing a tablet or capsule. Parents or carers should not give in to fractious children and not give medicines as then compliance may be a problem; at all stages, the child should be comforted and reassured. They must not be left with the impression that being given medicine is a punishment for being sick. Another problem is that the child may seem better, so parents/carers may not complete treatment, as with antibiotics.

The approach depends on the child's understanding and the circumstances:

- *Under 2 years*: Administration by parents if possible, using an approach which they believe is most likely to succeed.
- *2–5-year-olds* need a calm, gentle, firm and efficient approach after they have been told what is happening. Play and acting out may help them understand. Rewards may encourage further co-operation.
- *5–12-year-olds* also need encouragement, respect for their trust, and an explanation attuned to their understanding.
- *Over 12 years*. At this age children must have a proper understanding of what is happening and share in the decision making as well as the responsibility. They must feel in control.

What children and carers need to know

- The name of the medicine
- The reason for using it
- When and how to take it
- How to know if it is effective, and what to do if it is not
- What to do if one or more doses are missed
- How long to continue taking it
- The risks of stopping it early
- The most likely adverse effects; those unlikely, but important; and what to do if they occur
- Whether other medicines can be taken at the same time
- Whether other remedies alter the medicine's effect

Nursing staff involved with children need to be aware of medicine and dosage problems in children.

Dosing

Most doses of medicines have been derived from trials or from clinical experience and are usually given in terms of body weight as milligrams per kilogram of body weight (mg/kg). This assumes that the body weight is appropriate for the child's age, but this may not always be the case, since children grow at different rates and obesity is becoming more common. Before a dose is decided upon, the appropriateness of the child's weight for age and height should be assessed.

Alternatively, doses may be given for different age ranges as most drugs will have a wide safety margin (i.e. a large difference in the dose that produces a beneficial and toxic effect). For example, for paracetamol, the *BNF for Children* (2008) gives the following doses:

Oral paracetamol
Child 1–3 months: 30–60 mg every 8 hours
Child 3–12 months: 60–120 mg every 4–6 hours
Child 1–5 years: 120–250 mg every 4–6 hours
Child 6–12 years: 250–500 mg every 4–6 hours
Child 12–18 years: 500 mg every 4–6 hours

Once again, the appropriateness of the dose for the individual child, who may be small or large for their age, should also be assessed.

MAKE SURE THAT PAEDIATRIC
DOSES ARE CHECKED CAREFULLY

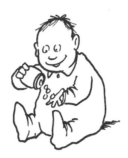

Using body surface area may be a more accurate method for dosing, as surface area better reflects developmental changes and function. However, determining surface area can be time-consuming and this method of dose calculation is generally reserved for potent drugs where there are small differences between effective and toxic doses (e.g. cytotoxic drugs).

Licensing and 'off-label' use

As stated earlier, many drugs are not tested in children which means that they are not specifically licensed for use in children. So although many medicines are licensed, they are often prescribed outside the terms of their Marketing Authorization (or licence) – known as 'off-label' prescribing – in relation to age, indication, dose of frequency, route of administration or formulation.

The Joint Royal College of Paediatrics and Child Health and the Neonatal and Paediatric Pharmacists Group (RCPH/NPPG) Standing Committee on Medicines has issued a policy statement:

- Those who prescribe for a child should choose the medicine which offers the best prospect of benefit for that child, with due regard to cost.
- The informed use of some unlicensed medicines or licensed medicines for unlicensed applications is necessary in paediatric practice.
- Health professionals should have ready access to sound information on any medicine they prescribe, dispense, or administer, and its availability.
- In general, it is not necessary to take additional steps beyond those taken when prescribing licensed medicines, to obtain the consent of parents, carers and child patients to prescribe or administer unlicensed medicines or licensed medicines for unlicensed applications.
- NHS Trusts and Health Authorities should support therapeutic practices that are advocated by a respectable, responsible body of professional opinion.

Nursing staff should be aware both when an unlicensed medicine is being administered and of their responsibilities.

Formulations

Appropriate formulations to enable administration of drugs to children are often not available. Children are often unable to swallow tablets or capsules, so liquid medicines are preferred. However, this is not always possible and crushing of tablets or manipulation of solid dosage forms into suspensions or powders is often required. (Always seek advice from pharmacy before doing this.)

Even parenteral medicines are usually only available in adult dose sizes. The strength of these products may mean that it is difficult to measure small doses for children and may lead to errors.

Some commercially available medicines may contain excipients that may cause adverse effects or be inappropriate to use in some children. Liquid preparations may contain excipients such as alcohol, sorbitol, propylene glycol or E-numbers; sugar-free medicines should be dispensed whenever possible. Parenteral products may contain benzyl alcohol or propylene glycol which can also cause adverse effects such as metabolic acidosis.

Problems associated with paediatric dosing

As well as changes in how the paediatric body handles drugs, doses may have to be adjusted for the following: fever, oedema, dehydration and GI disease. In these cases, the doctor should decide whether a dose needs to be adjusted.

In addition, there will be occasions when it will be difficult to give the dose required, because of the lack of an appropriate formulation – for example, to give 33 mg when only a 100 mg tablet is available. In these instances, it is advisable to contact the pharmacy department to see if a liquid preparation is available or can be prepared. If not, the doctor should be informed so that the dose can be modified, another drug can be prescribed, or another route can be used.

Another problem is frequency of dosing; dosing during the day will mean doses may have to be given at school which may not always be easy or possible. Medicines may have to be changed to those that can be given once or twice daily outside school hours.

References

British National Formulary for Children 2008 (BNF-C) (2008). Pharmaceutical Press, London.

I Costello, PF Long, IK Wong, C Tuleu and V Yeung. *Paediatric Drug Handling* (2007). Pharmaceutical Press, London.

DG Graheme-Smith and JK Aronson. *Oxford Textbook of Clinical Pharmacology and Drug Therapy* (2001). Oxford University Press, Oxford, 3rd ed.

Guy's, St. Thomas' and Lewisham Hospitals. *Paediatric Formulary* (2005). Guy's and St.Thomas' NHS Trust, London, 7th ed.

Royal College of Paediatrics and Child Health and Neonatal and Paediatric Pharmacists Group. *Medicines for Children 2003* (2003). RCPCH Publications Ltd, London, 2nd ed.

R Walker and C Whittlesea (editors). *Clinical Pharmacy and Therapeutics* (2007). Churchill Livingstone, Oxford, 4th ed.

USEFUL REFERENCE BOOKS

Neonatal Formulary: Drug Use in Pregnancy & the First Year of Life – current edition (latest edition = 5th, 2006). Northern Neonatal Network – Blackwell Publishing. Updates are available from: http://www.blackwellpublishing.com/medicine/bmj/nnf5/

British National Formulary for Children (BNF-C) – current edition (latest edition at time of writing is 2008). Pharmaceutical Press, London. Also available on-line at: http://bnfc. org/bnfc/

APPROXIMATE VALUES USEFUL IN THE CALCULATION OF DOSES IN CHILDREN

Table 11.3 gives average values for various parameters.

Table 11.3 Approximate values useful in the calculation of doses in children

AGE	WEIGHT kg	WEIGHT lb	HEIGHT cm	HEIGHT inch	SURFACE AREA (m²)	PERCENTAGE OF ADULT DOSE
Newborn	3.5*†¶	7.7*†¶	50*†¶	20*	0.23 or 0.24¶	12.5*†
1 month	4.2*¶	9*¶	55*¶	22*	0.26* or 0.27¶	14.5*
2 months	4.5*¶	10†	57¶	22	0.27† or 0.28¶	15*†
3 months	5.6*¶	12*	59*†	23*	0.32* or 0.33¶	18*
4 months	6.5*¶	14†	62*	24	0.34† or 0.36¶	20*†
6 months	7.7*¶	17*	67*¶	26*	0.40* or 0.41¶	22*
1 year	10*†¶	22*†	76*¶	30*	0.47*† or 0.49¶	25*†
3 years	15*†¶	33*†	94*¶	37*	0.62*† or 0.65¶	33* or 33.3†
5 years	18*¶	40*	108*¶	42*	0.73* or 0.74¶	40*
7 years	23*†¶	51*†	120*¶	47*	0.87¶ or 0.88*†	50*†
10 years	30*¶	66†	132¶	52	1.10¶	60†
12 years	39*†¶	86*†	148*¶	58*	1.25*† or 1.30¶	75*†
14 years	50*†¶	110†	163¶	64	1.50†¶	80†
16 years	58†	128†	167	67	1.65†	90†
ADULT						
Male	68*¶	150*	173*¶	68*	1.80*¶	
Female	56*¶	123*	163*¶	64*	1.60*¶	

* *Medicines for Children 2003*. RCPCH Publications Ltd, London, 2003.
† *Paediatric Formulary*. 7th ed. Guy's & St Thomas' NHS Trust. London 2005.
¶ *BNF for Children 2008*. BMJ Publishing Group, RPS Publishing, and RCPCH Publications, London 2008.

These values should only be used if a specific dose cannot be found, since they assumes the child is 'average'.

CALCULATING DOSAGES

When doing any calculation, you must make sure that the decimal point is in the right place. A difference of one place to the left or right could mean a 10-fold change in the dose, which could be fatal in some cases.

It is best to work in the smaller units, i.e. 100 micrograms as opposed to 0.1 milligrams. But even so, care must be taken with the number of noughts; a wrong dose can be fatal.

When calculating any dose, always get your answer checked.

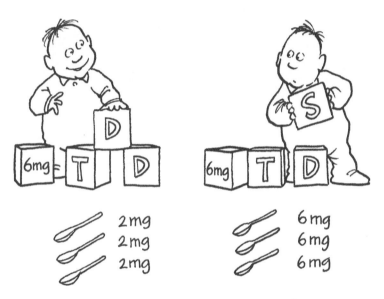

6mg T.D.D. = TOTAL DAILY DOSE OF 6mg

6mg T.D.S. = 6mg 'TER DIE SUMENDUS'
= 6mg THREE TIMES A DAY.

OBJECTIVES

At the end of this chapter, you should be familiar with the following:

- Drug handling in the elderly
- Specific problems in the elderly
- General principles

KEY POINTS

Prescribing in the Elderly

- As a person grows older it is almost inevitable that they will need some drug treatment.
- Changes in drug handling and response will occur.
  - The elderly are more prone to adverse reactions.
- The elderly will have more compliance issues.

Drug Handling and Drug Response

- Drug handling (pharmacokinetics) and drug response (pharmacodynamics) may change.
- Doses of some drugs may have to be reduced depending on how they are absorbed, broken down or metabolized, distributed or excreted.

General Principles

- A full medication history (including over-the-counter drugs) – this should highlight any previous adverse reaction, potential interactions and any compliance issues.
- Keep the regime simple – use as few drugs as possible.
- Clear and simple instructions should be given to the patient and the container must be clearly labelled. Various compliance aids are available, but it is important to establish that the patient can use them.
- Consider different formulations – e.g. liquids instead of large or small and fiddly tablets or capsules; combination products could reduce the number of medicines required; slow-release preparations to reduce adverse effects.
- If an elderly patient develops sudden symptoms or changes in behaviour or condition, consider if it could be drug related.
- Review medication regularly – do not continue to use a drug for longer than necessary.

INTRODUCTION

Approximately one-fifth of the population in England is over 60 years of age. This group receives 52 per cent of all prescriptions and often take a variety of drugs for several conditions. Of those aged over 75 years, 36 per cent are taking four or more drugs (polypharmacy).

As a person grows older, it is almost inevitable that drug treatment will be needed. A part of the ageing process will mean that physiological changes will occur that will affect how the elderly person handles and responds to drugs. They may also increase the risk of adverse effects and drug interactions.

DRUG HANDLING IN THE ELDERLY

Pharmacokinetics

Age-related changes in drug handling make older people more susceptible to drug effects.

Absorption

There is a reduction in gastric acid output and delay in gastric emptying with ageing. These changes do not significantly affect the absorption of the majority of drugs. Although the absorption of some drugs such as digoxin may be slower, the overall absorption is similar to that in the young.

Metabolism

A reduction in liver blood flow and in liver mass occurs as part of the ageing process; as a consequence, hepatic metabolism of some drugs may be altered. For those drugs eliminated primarily by liver metabolism, the capacity of the liver is reduced significantly by up to 60 per cent; resulting in decreased hepatic metabolism, increased plasma concentrations and longer half-lives, e.g. non-steroidal anti-inflammatory drugs (NSAIDs), antiepileptics and analgesics. The nutritional status of a person can also have a marked influence on the rate of drug metabolism. In frail elderly people, drug metabolism can be reduced to a greater extent than in elderly people with normal body weight.

Distribution

In older people, total body mass, lean body mass and total body water decrease, but total body fat increases. The effect of these changes on drug distribution depends on whether a dug is lipid- or water-soluble. A water-soluble drug is distributed mainly in the body water and lean body tissue. Because the elderly person has relatively less water and lean tissue, more of a water-soluble drug stays in the blood, which leads to increased blood concentration levels. As a result, a reduction in dose may be required. Examples include digoxin and gentamicin.

Since the elderly person has a higher proportion of body fat, more of a fat-soluble drug is distributed in the body fat. This can produce misleadingly low blood levels and may cause dosage to be incorrectly increased. The fatty tissue slowly releases stored drug into the bloodstream, and this explains why a fat-soluble sedative may produce a hangover effect. Examples include diazepam and lidocaine (lignocaine).

A decrease in albumin results in a reduction in the plasma protein binding of some drugs (e.g. phenytoin, warfarin). More non-bound drug is available to act at receptor sites and may result in toxicity. In these cases, a dose reduction may be necessary.

Renal excretion

The most important and predictable pharmacokinetic change seen in the elderly is a reduction in renal drug clearance.

Renal excretion is reduced because glomerular filtration rate, tubular secretion and renal blood flow are all reduced. Accumulation (due to increased blood levels) can occur if doses are not adjusted to account for the reduction in excretion by the kidneys. This decline in renal function can lead to an increase in adverse drug reactions, as glomerular filtration rate can decrease to around 50 mL/min by the age of 80. Drugs or those with active metabolites that are mainly excreted in the urine will need to be given at lower doses, particularly those with a narrow therapeutic index (e.g. warfarin, digoxin, lithium, phenytoin and carbamazepine). Tetracyclines are best avoided in the elderly because they can accumulate, causing nausea and vomiting, resulting in dehydration and further deterioration in renal function.

Disease states such as diabetes and heart failure can worsen renal function, as can an acute illness such as a chest infection that leads to dehydration.

Pharmacodynamics

The elderly appear to exhibit altered responses to drugs; in general, they have an increased sensitivity to drugs. This is due to probable changes in biomechanical responses, receptors, homeostatic changes and altered central nervous system (CNS) functions.

CNS changes may be significant – movement disorders may be due to neurotransmitter changes and increased confusion due to reduced cerebral blood flow. The brain shows increased sensitivity to certain drugs, e.g. benzodiazepines, opioids, anti-Parkinsonian drugs and antidepressants – even at normal doses – with the result that patients may become disoriented and confused.

When receptor changes are investigated in the elderly, beta-adrenergic receptors show a reduction in function and sensitivity, so agonist drugs such as salbutamol will have a reduced effect; propranolol (an antagonist) will also have a reduced effect.

Postural hypotension is common in the elderly. Orthostatic blood pressure control (control of blood pressure at rest and movement) is already impaired in the elderly, so they are more likely to suffer drug-induced hypotension, which can lead to dizziness and falls.

The thermoregulatory mechanisms may become impaired, which may lead to some degree of hypothermia, particularly drug-induced. This includes drugs that produce sedation, impaired subjective awareness of temperature, decreased mobility and muscular activity, and vasodilation. Commonly implicated drugs include phenothiazines, benzodiazepines, tricyclic antidepressants, opioids and alcohol, either on its own or with other drugs.

SPECIFIC PROBLEMS IN THE ELDERLY

Constipation

Constipation is a common problem in the elderly due to a decline in gastrointestinal motility as a result of ageing. Anticholinergic drugs, opiates, tricyclic antidepressants and antihistamines are more likely to cause constipation in the elderly.

Urological problems

Anticholinergic drugs may cause urinary retention in elderly men, especially those who have prostatic hypertrophy. Bladder instability is common in the elderly and urethral dysfunction more prevalent in elderly women. Loop diuretics may cause incontinence in such patients.

Psychotropic drugs

Hypnotics with long half-lives are a significant problem and can cause daytime drowsiness, unsteadiness from impaired balance, and confusion. Short-acting ones may also be problematic and should only be used for short periods if essential.

The elderly are more sensitive to benzodiazepines than the young; the mechanism of this increased sensitivity is not known – smaller doses should be used. Tricyclic antidepressants can cause postural hypotension and confusion in the elderly.

Warfarin

The elderly are more sensitive to warfarin; doses can be about 25 per cent less than in younger people. This phenomenon may be due to age-related changes in pharmacodynamic factors. The exact mechanism is unknown.

Digoxin

The elderly appear to be more sensitive to the adverse effects of digoxin, but not to the cardiac effects. Factors include potassium loss (which increases cell sensitivity to digoxin) due to diuretics and reduced renal excretion.

Diuretics

The elderly can easily lose too much fluid and become dehydrated and this can affect treatment of hypotension. Diurectics can also cause extra potassium loss (hypokalaemia) which may increase the effects of digoxin and hence contribute to digoxin toxicity. The elderly can be more prone to gout because of diuretics' side effect of uric acid retention (hyperuricaemia).

Compliance

Compliance can be a problem in the elderly as complicated drug regimes may be difficult for them to follow; they may stop taking the drugs or take wrong doses at the wrong time. Dispensing drugs for elderly and confused people can be made easier by using various compliance aids. These are devices in which medication is dispensed for patients who experience difficulty in taking their medicines, particularly those who have difficulty in co-ordinating their medication regime or have large number of medicines to take. They have compartments for each day of the week and each compartment is divided into four sections, i.e. morning, lunch, dinner, bedtime. They do not provide benefit to all types of patients and are not useful for patients who have visual impairment, dexterity problems or severe cognitive impairment.

Adverse reactions

An adverse reaction to a drug is likely to be two or three times more common in the elderly than in other patients. There are several reasons for this:

- Elderly patients often need several drugs at the same time and there is a close relationship between the number of drugs taken and the incidence of adverse reactions.
- Pharmacokinetics in the elderly (how they handle drugs) may be impaired so that they may experience higher concentrations of some drugs unless the dose is suitably adjusted.
- Drugs that are associated with adverse reactions, such as digoxin, diuretics, NSAIDs, hypotensives and various centrally acting agents, are often prescribed for elderly patients.

GENERAL PRINCIPLES

Often, older people have problems with the practicalities of taking medicines and have compliance issues. In addition, people who are confused, depressed or have poor memories may have difficulty in taking medicines. The following general principles may be helpful:

- A full medication history (including over-the-counter drugs) – this should highlight any previous adverse reaction, potential interactions and any compliance issues.
- Keep the regime simple – use as few drugs as possible.
- Clear and simple instructions should be given to the patient and the container must be clearly labelled. Many older people are unable to read leaflets and labels due to failing eyesight, and may need specially written instructions.
- Various compliance aids are available, but it is important to establish that the patient can use them.
- Consider different formulations – liquids instead of large or small and fiddly tablets or capsules; combination products to reduce the number of medicines to take; slow-release preparations to reduce adverse effects.
- If an elderly patient develops sudden symptoms or changes in behaviour or condition, consider if it could be drug related.
- Review medication regularly – do not continue to use a drug for longer than necessary.

References

Anon. Prescribing for the older person. *MeReC Bulletin* 2000; **11** (10): 37–40.

D Armour and C Cairns. *Medicines in the Elderly* (2002). Pharmaceutical Press, London.

G Downie, J Mackenzie and A Williams. *Pharmacology and Medicines Management for Nurses* (2008). Churchill Livingstone, Edinburgh, 4th ed.

DG Graheme-Smith and JK Aronson. *Oxford Textbook of Clinical Pharmacology and Drug Therapy* (2001). Oxford University Press, Oxford, 3rd ed.

B Greenstein and D Gould. *Trounce's Clinical Pharmacology for Nurses* (2004). Churchill Livingstone, Edinburgh, 17th ed.

R Walker and C Whittlesea (editors). *Clinical Pharmacy and Therapeutics* (2007). Churchill Livingstone, Oxford, 4th ed.

13 SOURCES AND INTERPRETATION OF DRUG INFORMATION

OBJECTIVES

At the end of this chapter, you should be familiar with the following:

- Sources of drug information
- Summary of product characteristics (SPC)

KEY POINTS

Sources of Drug Information

General

- *British National Formulary* (BNF) – website: http://www.bnf.org/bnf/
- *British National Formulary for Children* (BNFC) – website: http://bnfc.org/bnfc/
- *Electronic Medicines Compendium* – information provided by drug companies of their products – website: http://emc.medicines.org.uk/

Specialist books

- *Neonatal Formulary: Drug Use in Pregnancy & the First Year of Life* – current edition
- *Paediatric Formulary* – Guy's, St Thomas' and Lewisham Hospitals
- *Injectable Medicines Administration Guide* – Pharmacy Department, UCL Hospitals – Blackwell Publishing

Summary of Product Characteristics (SPC)

Information can be supplied by drug manufacturers in the form of a drug data sheet or summary of product characteristics (SPC). It provides essential information to ensure that the drug or medicine is used correctly, effectively and safely.

The information given in the SPC is also summarized in the package insert found inside the box. The package insert contains the basic information necessary for the administration and monitoring of the drug.

INTRODUCTION

Before administering any drug, you should have some idea of how that drug acts, its effect on the body and possible adverse effects. This is particularly true when dealing with parenteral products as they will have a more immediate and dramatic effect than oral preparations.

Basic drug information can be found in reference books or, increasingly, from web-based resources; many of the text-based resources are now also available on-line.

The following is a list of some sources of drug information. It is not meant to be exhaustive, but a list of resources that should be readily available on the ward, either as a book or via the Internet. The paediatric books should be available on paediatric wards; if not, they will be available in the hospital pharmacy.

SOURCES OF DRUG INFORMATION

General

- *British National Formulary* (BNF) – current edition
  (Latest edition = No. 57, March 2009)
  Website: http://www.bnf.org/bnf/
- *British National Formulary for Children* (BNFC) – current edition
  (Latest edition = 2008)
  Website: http://bnfc.org/bnfc/
- *Electronic Medicines Compendium* – information provided by drug companies of their products.
  Website: http://emc.medicines.org.uk/
- Drug package insert – if the drug is available in its original container, then there should be a package insert containing general information for that drug.

Specialist books

- *Neonatal Formulary: Drug Use in Pregnancy & the First Year of Life* – current edition (Latest edition = 5th, 2006)
  Northern Neonatal Network – Blackwell Publishing
  Updates are available from: http://www.blackwellpublishing.com/medicine/bmj/nnf5/
- *Paediatric Formulary* – current edition (Latest edition = 7th, 2005)
  Guy's, St Thomas' and Lewisham Hospitals

Your local hospital pharmacy department will be able to give advice on any aspects of dosing and administration of drugs.

Injectable Medicines Administration Guide – 2nd edition (2007). Pharmacy Departmnt, UCL Hospitals – Blackwell Publishing.

SUMMARY OF PRODUCT CHARACTERISTICS (SPC)

Before a drug is marketed, it is extensively researched and tested over many years. During this time, a great deal of information is gathered about efficacy, side effects and toxicology.

The most important information regarding the drug is documented in the Summary of Product Characteristics – the SPC, also called the data sheet – which is officially approved when the medicine is licensed for use. These can be viewed via the *Electronic Medicines Compendium* website (see list of Sources of Drug Information).

The main purpose of an SPC is to provide essential information to ensure that the drug or medicine is used correctly, effectively and safely.

What an SPC contains

All SPCs are presented in the same way, using a standard heading for each section. In the following list you will find a brief description of each of these headings.

1. Trade name of the medicinal product
The brand name of the drug or medicine.

2. Qualitative and quantitative composition
The generic or chemical names of the active ingredients and the amount of each active ingredient, e.g. amount per tablet, amount per volume of solution.

3. Pharmaceutical form
The form in which the medicine is presented, e.g. tablets, suppositories, ointment.

4. Clinical particulars
How the medicine should be used; includes information for prescribers to ensure that patients are treated appropriately, taking into account the patient's medical history, any co-existing diseases or conditions and other current treatments.

4.1 Therapeutic indications
The diseases or conditions that the medicine is licensed to treat.

4.2 Posology and method of administration
Posology refers to the science of dosage, i.e. how much of a medicine should be given to a patient. The dose of the drug is given, including any changes in dose that may be necessary according to age or co-existing disease or condition, such as renal or hepatic impairment. Where relevant, information is also given on the timing of doses in relation to meals.

The maximum single dose, the maximum daily dose and the maximum dose for a course of treatment may also be given.

4.3 Contra-indications
Anything about a patient's condition, medical history or current treatments that may indicate that this medicine should not be given.

4.4 Special warnings and special precautions for use
Any circumstances or condition where the drug should be used with particular care.

4.5 Interactions with other medicaments and other forms of interaction

Any other medicines, or anything else that the patient is likely to take, which may react with the drug, for example, food or alcohol as well as other drugs.

4.6 Pregnancy and lactation

Advice on the risks associated with using the drug at various stages of pregnancy and in fertile women, based upon the results of animal studies and any published observations in humans. If the drug or any of its metabolites is excreted in breast milk, the probability and nature of any adverse effects in the infant are described, and whether breast feeding should continue or not.

4.7 Effects on ability to drive and use machines

Whether or not the medicine is likely to impair a patient's ability to drive or operate machinery and if so, the extent of the effect.

4.8 Undesirable effects

A description of the adverse effects which may occur, including how likely they are to happen, how severe they may be and for how long they are likely to last.

4.9 Overdose

A description of the signs and symptoms of overdose, together with advice on how to treat.

5. Pharmacological properties

Information about how the medicine works and how it is handled by the body.

5.1 Pharmacodynamic properties

How the medicine achieves, or is believed to achieve, its therapeutic effect in the body.

5.2 Pharmacokinetic properties

Information on how the medicine is taken up, distributed in the body and then removed.

Where appropriate, additional information may be included as to how the pharmacokinetics may change according to, for example, the patient's age or state of health.

5.3 Preclinical safety data

Describes the effects of the drug that were observed in studies before being used in humans, which could be of relevance to the prescriber in assessing the risks and benefits of treatment.

6. Pharmaceutical particulars

Information on the medicine ingredients, storage and packaging.

6.1 List of excipients

The contents of the medicine apart from the active ingredients, such as binding agents, solvents and flavourings are given.

6.2 Incompatibilities

In addition to the information given under 'Interaction with other medicaments and other forms of interaction', any other medicines or materials that interact with the drug and with which it should therefore not be used or mixed.

6.3 Shelf life

The maximum length of time for which the medicine may be stored under the specified conditions stated and after which it should not be used.

6.4 Special precautions for storage

The conditions in which the medicine must be stored to avoid degradation, for example, by excessive temperatures or light.

6.5 Nature and contents of container

Description of the packaging and any other materials included in the pack, such as desiccants, are given.

6.6 Instructions for use/handling

Instructions for the preparation or administration of the medicine in addition to those given under 'Posology and method of administration'.

7. Marketing authorization holder

The drug company holding the marketing authorization granted by the licensing authority.

8. Marketing authorization number

The licence number for the marketing authorization granted by the licensing authority.

9. Date of first authorization/renewal of authorization

The date when the marketing authorization was first granted. If the licence has at some time been suspended, the date when the licence was renewed.

10. Date of (partial) revision of the text

The last date on which an alteration to the wording of the SPC was officially made to reflect, for example, the addition of a new therapeutic indication or a change in the pack sizes available.

The information given in the SPC is also summarized in the package insert found inside the box.

The package insert contains the basic information necessary for the administration and monitoring of the drug. This is particularly useful when administering parenteral drugs as it gives information on dosing, diluents, rate of administration, etc. The following is the package insert for clarithromycin injection (Klaricid®).

TECHNICAL LEAFLET
KLARICID® I.V.
500 mg clarithromycin

Presentation
Klaricid IV is a sterile freeze-dried powder form of clarithromycin. Each vial is a single dose of clarithromycin and contains: 500 mg Clarithromycin, Lactobionic Acid, Sodium Hydroxide, and Nitrogen.
Details of the preparation of suitable solutions for IV administration are given in the section on Administration.

Actions
Clarithromycin is an anti-bacterial agent. It is a semi-synthetic derivative of erythromycin A.

Uses
For the treatment of infections caused by susceptible organisms, whenever parenteral therapy is required, e.g. upper and lower respiratory tract infections and skin and soft tissue infections.

Contra-indications
Known hypersensitivity to macrolide antibiotic drugs. Concomitant administration of clarithromycin and any of the following drugs is contra-indicated: cisapride, pimozide, terfenadine, and ergot derivatives. Similar effects seen with astemizole.

Precautions
Caution in administering to patients with impaired hepatic and renal function. Prolonged or repeated use of clarithromycin may result in an overgrowth of non-susceptible bacteria or fungi. The use of clarithromycin in patients concurrently taking drugs metabolized by the cytochrome p450 system may be associated with elevations in serum levels of these other drugs.

Interactions
No interaction with oral contraceptives. Drugs metabolized by the cytochrome p450 system (e.g. warfarin, ergot alkaloids, triazolam, midazolam, disopyramide, lovastatin, rifabutin, phenytoin, cilostazol, methylprednisolone, quinidine, sildenafil, alprazolam, vinblastine, valproate, cyclosporin, and tacrolimus). Rhabdomyolysis co-incident with the co-administration of clarithromycin and HMG-CoA reductase inhibitors, such as lovastatin and simvastatin, has been reported.
There have been post-marketing reports of colchicine toxicity with concomitant use of clarithromycin and colchicines, especially in the elderly, some of which occurred in patients with renal insufficiency.
Theophylline, warfarin. (Prothrombin time should be frequently monitored in these patients.)
Digoxin, quinidine, disopyramide. (Monitoring of serum digoxin, quinidine, disopyramide levels should be considered.)
Carbamazepine.
Ritonavir, for patients with renal impairment, dosage adjustments should be considered: CL_{CR} 30 to 60 mL/min, reduce dose by 50%; CL_{CR} <30 mL/min, reduce dose by 75%.
Doses of clarithromycin greater than 1 g/day should not be coadministered with ritonavir.

Fig 13.1 Package insert for Klaricid®

Side Effects

Commonest side effects seen at the injection site, e.g. inflammation, tenderness, phlebitis and pain. Others including nausea, vomiting, diarrhoea, paraesthesia, dyspepsia, abdominal pain, headache, tooth and tongue discolouration, arthralgia, myalgia and allergic reactions ranging from urticaria and mild skin eruptions and angioedema to anaphylaxis, have been reported. There have been reports of Stevens-Johnson syndrome/ toxic epidermal necrolysis with orally administered clarithromycin. Stomatitis, glossitis and oral monilia have been reported. Alteration of the sense of smell, usually in conjunction with taste perversion has also been reported with oral treatment. There have been reports of transient central nervous system side-effects including dizziness, vertigo, anxiety, insomnia, bad dreams, tinnitus, confusion, disorientation, hallucinations, psychosis and depersonalisation. There have been reports of hearing loss with clarithromycin which is usually reversible upon withdrawal of therapy. There have been rare reports of hypoglycaemia, some of which have occurred in patients on concomitant oral hypoglycaemic agents or insulin. There have been very rare reports of reversible uveitis, mainly in patients on concomitant rifabutin. Pseudomembranous colitis has been reported rarely with clarithromycin and may range in severity from mild to life threatening. Isolated cases of leukopenia and thrombocytopenia have been reported. Hepatic dysfunction, including altered liver function tests, cholestasis with or without jaundice and hepatitis, has been reported. Cases of increased serum creatinine, interstitial nephritis and renal failure, pancreatitis and convulsions have been reported rarely. As with other macrolides, QT prolongation, ventricular tachycardia and Torsade de Pointes have been rarely reported with clarithromycin. There have been reports of colchicine toxicity with concomitant use of clarithromycin and colchicines; deaths have been reported in such patients.

If any other undesirable effect occurs, which is not mentioned above, the patient should be advised to give details to his/her doctor.

Use In Pregnancy and Lactating Women

Klaricid should not be used during pregnancy or lactation unless the clinical benefit is considered to outweigh the risk. Clarithromycin has been found in the milk of lactating animals and in human breast milk.

Recommended Dosage

Intravenous therapy may be given for 2 to 5 days and should be changed to oral clarithromycin therapy when appropriate.

Adults: The recommended dosage of Klaricid IV is 1.0 gram daily, divided into two 500 mg doses, appropriately diluted as described below.

Children: At present, there are insufficient data to recommend a dosage regime for routine use in children.

Elderly: As for adults.

Renal Impairment: In patients with renal impairment who have creatinine clearance less than 30 mL/min, the dosage of clarithromycin should be reduced to one half of the normal recommended dose.

Recommended Administration

Clarithromycin should not be given as a bolus or an intramuscular injection.

Klaricid IV should be administered into one of the larger proximal veins as an IV infusion over 60 minutes, using a solution concentration of about 2 mg/mL.

Fig 13.1 *Continued*

STEP 1

Add 10 ml sterilized Water for Injections into the vial and shake.
Use within 24 hours.
May be stored from 5°C up to room temperature.

DO NOT USE
- Diluents containing preservatives
- Diluents containing inorganic salts

STEP 2

Add 10 mL from Step 1 to 250 mL of a suitable diluent (see below).
This provides a 2 mg/mL solution.
Use within 6 hours (at room temperature) or within 24 hours if stored at 5°C.

DO NOT USE
- Solution strengths greater than 2 mg/mL (0.2%)
- Rapid infusion rates (< 60 minutes)
- Failure to observe these precautions may result in pain along the vein.

Recommended Diluents
5% dextrose in Lactated Ringer's Solution, 5% dextrose, Lactated Ringer's solution, 5% dextrose in 0.3% sodium chloride, Normosol-M in 5% dextrose, Normosol-R in 5% dextrose, 5% dextrose in 0.45% sodium chloride, or 0.9% sodium chloride. Compatibility with other IV additives has not been established.

Overdosage
There is no experience of overdosage after IV administration of clarithromycin. However, reports indicate that the ingestion of large amounts of clarithromycin orally can be expected to produce gastrointestinal symptoms. Adverse reactions accompanying oral overdosage should be treated by gastric lavage and supportive measures.
As with other macrolides, clarithromycin serum levels are not expected to be appreciably affected by haemodialysis or peritoneal dialysis.
One patient who had a history of bipolar disorder ingested 8 g of clarithromycin and showed altered mental status, paranoid behaviour, hypokalaemia and hypoxaemia.

Storage
Can be stored at up to 30°C. Store in the original container as the powder is sensitive to light. See carton and vial for expiry date. The product should not be used after this date.

Product Licence Number
0037/0251

Legal Category
POM
Marketed in the UK by: Abbott Laboratories Ltd., Queenborough, Kent, ME11 5EL
Date of preparation of leaflet: May 1999. Revised: September 2006.

100-606-201

Fig 13.1 *Continued*

Let us look at the Klaricid® package insert in more detail as this is the usual form in which drug information will be presented you. The important points to note would be the dosing information, the administration information and recommended dilutents.

Dosing information

Recommended Dosage
Intravenous therapy may be given for 2 to 5 days and should be changed to oral clarithromycin therapy when appropriate.

Adults: The recommended dosage of Klaricid IV is 1.0 gram daily, divided into two 500 mg doses, appropriately diluted as described below.

Children: At present, there are insufficient data to recommend a dosage regime for routine use in children.

Elderly: As for adults.

Renal Impairment: In patients with renal impairment who have creatinine clearance less than 30mL/min, the dosage of clarithromycin should be reduced to one half of the normal recommended dose.

Fig 13.2 Klaricid® dosing information

- The normal dose for adults (including the elderly) is 500 mg twice a day for 2–5 days.
- In patients with renal impairment, the dose may have to be reduced.
- Clarithromycin is not recommended in children.

Administration information

Recommended Administration
<u>Clarithromycin should not be given as a bolus or an intramuscular injection.</u>
Klaricid IV should be administered into one of the larger proximal veins as an IV infusion over 60 minutes, using a solution concentration of about 2mg/mL.

STEP 1

Add 10mL sterilized Water for Injections into the vial and shake.
Use within 24 hours.
May be stored from 5°C up to room temperature.

STEP 2

Add 10mL from Step 1 to 250mL of a suitable diluent (see below).
This provides a 2mg/mL solution.
Use within 6 hours (at room temperature) or within 24 hours if stored at 5°C.

DO NOT USE
- Diluents containing preservatives
- Diluents containing inorganic salts

DO NOT USE
- Solution strengths greater than 2mg/mL (0.2%)
- Rapid infusion rates (< 60 mins)
- Failure to observe these precautions may result in pain along the vein.

Fig 13.3 Klaricid® administration information

Administration

- Clarithromycin should **not** be given as a IV bolus or by IM injection – it must be given as an intermittent infusion.
- The infusion must be given over at least 60 minutes.
- The concentration of the infusion should not be greater than 2 mg/mL (0.2%); usually given in 250 mL of diluent.
  Let us see how this is calculated:
  Maximum concentration is 2 mg/mL, which is equal to:

$$1 \text{ mg in } \frac{1}{2} \text{mL} = 0.5 \text{ mL}$$

Therefore, for a 500 mg dose: $500 \times 0.5 = 250$ mL
So, the minimum volume for a 500 mg dose would be 250 mL.

Reconstitution information

- Water for Injections BP must be used.
- The volume for reconstitution is 10 mL.
- Once reconstituted, it must be used within 24 hours.
- Once added to the infusion bag, it must be used within 6 hours (24 hours if stored in a fridge).

Recommended diluents

Recommended Diluents
5% dextrose in Lactated Ringer's Solution, 5% dextrose, Lactated Ringer's solution, 5% dextrose in 0.3% sodium chloride, Normosol-M in 5% dextrose, Normosol-R in 5% dextrose, 5% dextrose in 0.45% sodium chloride, or 0.9% sodium chloride. Compatibility with other IV additives has not been established.

Fig 13.4 Recomended diluents for Klaricid®

Suitable infusion fluids include: sodium chloride 0.9% or 5% dextrose.

Other points to note

- **Contra-indications**: hypersensitivity to clarithromycin, otherwise nothing else of note.
- **Precautions**: caution in administering to patients with impaired hepatic and renal function.
- **Incompatibilities**: this information would be useful if several drugs are being given parenterally and going through the same IV line or mixed in the same infusion bag. In this case, nothing is reported.
- **Side effects**: the most commonly seen side effects are those seen at the injection site, e.g. inflammation, tenderness, phlebitis and pain.

The purpose of this revision test is to test your ability at drug calculations after you have finished working through the book.

You should get most, if not all, of the questions right. If you get the wrong answers for any particular section, then you should go back and re-do that section, as it indicates that you have not fully understood that type of calculation.

BASICS

The aim of this section is see if you understand basic principles such as fractions, decimals, powers and using calculators.

Long multiplication
Solve the following:

1 567×405
2 265×2.45

Long division
Solve the following:

3 $4158 \div 21$
4 $26.88 \div 1.12$

Fractions
Solve the following, leaving your answers as fractions:

5 $\dfrac{15}{16} \times \dfrac{4}{7}$

6 $\dfrac{4}{9} \times \dfrac{2}{3}$

7 $\dfrac{3}{8} \div \dfrac{6}{7}$

8 $\dfrac{2}{5} \div \dfrac{12}{15}$

Convert each of the following fractions to a decimal (give answers to 2 decimal places):

9 $\dfrac{4}{7}$

10 $\dfrac{8}{18}$

Decimals

Solve the following:

11 2.15×0.64
12 $4.2 \div 0.125$
13 2.6×100
14 $45.67 \div 1,000$

Convert the following decimals to fractions:

15 0.4
16 0.025

Roman numerals

Write the following as ordinary numbers:

17 III
18 VII

Powers

Convert the following to a proper number:

19 2.3×10^2

Convert the following number to a power of 10:

20 800,000

PER CENT AND PERCENTAGES

This section is designed to see if you understand the concept of per cent and percentages.

21 How much is 34% of 500 g?
22 What percentage is 220 g of 500 g?

UNITS AND EQUIVALENCES

This section is designed to re-test your knowledge of units and how to convert from one unit to another.
   Convert the following amounts.

Units of weight

23 0.125 milligrams (mg) to micrograms (mcg)
24 0.5 grams (g) to milligrams (mg)
25 250 nanograms (ng) to micrograms (mcg)

Units of volume

26 0.45 litres (L) to millilitres (mL)

Units of amount of substance

27 0.15 moles (mol) to millimoles (mmol)

DRUG STRENGTHS OR CONCENTRATIONS

This section is designed to see if you understand the various ways in which drug strengths can be expressed.

Percentage concentration

28 How much glucose (in grams) is there in a 500 mL infusion of glucose 10%?

mg/mL concentrations

29 What is the concentration (in mg/mL) of a 30% sodium chloride ampoule?

'1 in ...' concentrations or ratio strengths

30 You have a 1 mL ampoule of adrenaline/epinephrine 1 in 1,000. How much adrenaline/epinephrine – in milligrams – does the ampoule contain?

Parts per million (ppm) strengths

31 If a disinfectant solution contains 1,000 ppm of chlorine, how much chlorine (in grams) would be present in 5 litres?

DOSAGE CALCULATIONS

This section tests you on the type of calculations you will be doing every day on the ward. It includes dosages based on patient parameters and paediatric calculations.

Calculating the number of tablets or capsules required

The strength of the tablets or capsules you have available does not always correspond to the dose required. Therefore you have to be able to calculate the number of tablets or capsules needed.

32 Dose prescribed is lisinopril 15 mg. You have lisinopril 5 mg tablets available. How many tablets do you need?

Drug dosage

Sometimes the dose is given on a body weight basis or in terms of body surface area. The following questions test your ability to calculate doses on these parameters.

Work out the dose required for the following:

33 Dose = 7.5 mg/kg   Weight = 78 kg
34 Dose = 4 mcg/kg/min   Weight = 56 kg
35 Dose = 4.5 mg/m^2 Surface area = 1.94 m^2

(Give your answer to 3 decimal places.)

Calculating dosages

Calculate how much drug you need (in mL) for the following dosages:

36 You have haloperidol injection 5 mg in 1 mL; amount required = 6 mg
37 You have diazepam suspension 2 mg in 5 mL; amount required = 5 mg
38 You have codeine phosphate syrup 25 mg in 5 mL; amount required = 30 mg
39 You have co-trimoxazole injection 480 mg in 5 mL ampoules; amount required = 2,040 mg
What volume and how many ampoules do you need?

Paediatric calculations

40 The dose of morphine for a 6-month-old child (7 kg) is 200 mcg/kg. How much do you need to draw up if morphine is available in a 10 mg/mL ampoule?

Other factors to take into account are displacement volumes for antibiotic injections.

41 A child is prescribed co-amoxiclav injection at a dose of 350 mg. The displacement volume for co-amoxiclav is 0.9 mL per 1.2 g vial. How much Water for Injections do you need to add to ensure a strength of 1.2 g per 20 mL?

MOLES AND MILLIMOLES

This section is designed to see if you understand the concept of millimoles. Millimoles are used to describe the 'amount of substance', and are usually the units for body electrolytes (e.g. sodium 138 mmol/L).

Moles and millimoles

42 Approximately how many millimoles of sodium are there in a 200 mL infusion of sodium bicarbonate 8.4%? (Molecular mass of sodium bicarbonate = 84)

Molarity

43 How many grams of sodium chloride is required to make 100 ml of a 0.6 M solution? (Molecular mass of sodium chloride = 58.5)

INFUSION RATE CALCULATIONS

This section tests your knowledge of various infusion rate calculations. It is designed to see if you know the different drop factors for different giving sets and fluids, as well as being able to convert volumes to drops and vice versa.

Calculation of drip rates

44 What is the drip rate required to give 1 litre of sodium chloride 0.9% infusion over 8 hours using a standard giving set?

45 What is the drip rate required to give 1 unit of blood (500 mL) over 6 hours using a standard giving set?

Conversion of dosages to mL/hour

Sometimes it may be necessary to convert a dose (mg/min) to an infusion rate (mL/hour).

46 You have an infusion of dobutamine 250 mg in 250 mL. The dose required is 6 mcg/kg/min and the patient weighs 77 kg. What is the rate in mL/hour?

47 You are required to give a patient glyceryl trinitrate (50 mg in 50 mL) as a continuous infusion at a rate of 50 micrograms/min. At what is the rate should the infusion pump be set (mL/hour)?

Conversion of mL/hour back to a dose

48 You have enoximone 100 mg in 100 mL and the rate at which the pump is running is 30 mL/hour. What dose is the pump delivering? (Patient's weight = 96 kg)

Calculating the length of time for IV infusions

49 A 1 litre infusion of sodium chloride 0.9% is being given at a rate of 28 drops/min (SGS).
How long will the infusion run at the specified rate?

50 A 500 mL infusion of glucose 5% is being given at a rate of 167 mL/hour. How long will the infusion run at the specified rate?

COMPARE YOUR SCORES

Check your answers below and compare with your result from the pre test.

	MARK OUT OF 50	PERCENTAGE SCORE (double the figure in the previous column.)	DIFFERENCE (Subtract the revision % score from the pre-test % score in the previous column.)
Pre-test score			
Revision test score			

ANSWERS TO REVISION TEST

Basics

Long multiplication
1 229,635
2 649.25

Long division
3 198
4 24

Fractions

5 $\dfrac{5}{28}$

6 $\dfrac{8}{27}$

7 $\dfrac{7}{16}$

8 $\dfrac{1}{2}$

9 0.57
10 0.44

Decimals
11 1.376
12 33.6
13 260
14 0.04567

15 $\dfrac{2}{5}$

16 $\dfrac{1}{40}$

Roman numerals
17 3
18 7

Powers
19 230
20 8×10^5

Per cent and percentages
21 170 g
22 44%

Units and equivalences

Units of weight
23 125 micrograms
24 500 milligrams
25 0.25 micrograms

Units of volume
26 450 millilitres

Units of amount of substance
27 150 millimoles

Drug strengths or concentrations

Percentage concentration
28 50 g

mg/mL concentrations
29 300 mg/mL

'1 in ...' concentrations or ratio strengths
30 1 mg

Parts per million (ppm) strengths
31 5 g

Dosage calculations

Calculating the number of tablets or capsules required
32 Three lisinopril 5 mg tablets

Drug dosage
33 585 mg
34 224 micrograms/min
35 8.730 mg

Calculating dosages
36 1.2 mL
37 12.5 mL
38 6 mL
39 21.25 mL; 5 ampoules

Paediatric calculations
40 0.14 mL
41 19.1 mL

Moles, millimoles and molarity

Moles and millimoles
42 200 mmol sodium

Molarity
43 3.51 g sodium chloride

Infusion rate calculations

Calculation of drip rates
44 41.7 drops/min (rounded to 42 drops/min)
45 20.8 drops/min (rounded to 21 drops/min)

Conversion of dosages to mL/hour
46 27.7 mL/hour
47 3 mL/hour

Conversion of mL/hour back to a dose
48 5.21 mcg/kg/min (approx. 5 mcg/kg/min)

Calculating the length of time for IV infusions
49 11.90 hours (approx. 12 hours)
50 2.99 hours (approx. 3 hours)

Answers to problems

Here you will find the answers to the problems set in each chapter:

Chapter 3 Per cent and percentages

Question 1   927
Question 2   35,973
Question 3   450
Question 4   48.36
Question 5   50.008 (50)
Question 6   8%
Question 7   84%
Question 8   63%
Question 9   28%
Question 10 33.8% (to 1 decimal place)

Chapter 4 Units and equivalences

Question 1   Answer: 12.5 grams

kg			g	
0	0	1	2	5
	1	*2*	*3*	

The decimal point goes between the 2 and the 5.

Question 2   Answer: 0.25 micrograms

mcg			ng
0	2	5	0
	3	*2*	*1*

The decimal point goes between the 0 and the 2.

Question 3   Answer: 3,200 millilitres

L			ml
3	2	0	0
	1	*2*	*3*

The decimal point goes after the final 0.

Question 4   Answer: 27.3 millimoles

mol			mmol	
0	0	2	7	3
	1	*2*	*3*	

The decimal point goes between the 7 and the 3.

Question 5   Answer: 3.75 kilograms

kg	←		g
3	7	5	0
	3	2	1

The decimal point goes between the 3 and the 7.

Question 6   Answer: 50,000 micrograms

g	→	mg	→			mcg
0	0	5	0	0	0	0
	1	2	3	1	2	3

As we are going from grams to micrograms, this is the same as two separate conversions. So the decimal point must move twice, i.e. 6 places (3 and 3).

The decimal point goes after the final zero.

Question 7   Answer: 0.025 kilograms

kg	←		g	←		mg
0	0	2	5	0	0	0
	3	2	1	3	2	1

As we are going from milligrams to kilograms, this is the same as two separate conversions. So the decimal point must move twice, i.e. 6 places (3 and 3).

The decimal point goes between the two zeros.

Question 8   Answer: 4,500 nanograms

The 10^{-6} is a power. The −6 indicates that it is a negative power, i.e. the number is divided by 10 six times.

Practically speaking, we move the decimal point six places to the left, i.e.

$$4.5 \times 10^{-6}\,g = 0.0000045\,g$$

When converting from a larger unit to a smaller unit, you multiply by 1,000.

Thus for each conversion, multiply by 1,000, i.e. move the decimal point three places to the right:

$$0.0000045\,g = 0.0045\,mg = 4.5\ \text{micrograms}$$
$$= 4,500\ \text{nanograms}$$

You could also use the boxes method. As the number is divided by 10 six times, this would mean 5 zeros before the 4 (don't forget that the decimal point is originally after the [4.5], so this means that it goes between the fifth and sixth zero):

g	→	mg	→	mcg	→	ng
0	0	0	0	0	0	4	5	0	0
.	1	2	3	1	2	3	1	2	3

As we are going from grams to nanograms, this is the same as **three** separate conversions. So the decimal point must move three times, i.e. 9 places (3 and 3 and 3).

The decimal point goes after the final zero to give the answer 4500 nanograms.

Question 9   **Answer:** 500 micrograms digoxin in 2 mL

First convert milligrams to micrograms. You are going from a larger unit to a smaller unit; so you multiply by 1,000 to remove the decimal point:

$$0.25 \times 1,000 = 250 \text{ micrograms}$$

Thus you have 250 micrograms in 1 mL.
Multiply by 2 to find out how much is in 2 mL, i.e.

$$250 \times 2 = 500 \text{ microgram}$$

Question 10   **Answer:** 100 micrograms fentanyl in a 2 mL ampoule

First convert milligrams to micrograms to remove the decimal point: you are going from a larger unit to a smaller unit; so multiply by 1,000:

$$0.05 \times 1,000 = 50 \text{ micrograms}$$

Thus you have 50 micrograms in 1 mL. To find out how much there will be in a 2 mL ampoule, multiply by 2:

$$50 \text{ micrograms} \times 2 = 100 \text{ micrograms}$$

OR USING BOXES

mg	→	mcg
0	0	5	0
	1	2	3

The decimal point goes at the end; thus you have 50 micrograms in 1 mL.

To find out how much is in a 2 mL ampoule, multiply by 2:

$$50 \text{ micrograms} \times 2 = 100 \text{ micrograms}$$

Chapter 5 Drug strengths or concentrations

Question 1	0.9 g in 100 mL
	9 g in 1,000 mL
	Answer: 9 g
Question 2	Potassium 0.3 g in 100 mL
	3 g in 1,000 mL
	Sodium 0.18 g in 100 mL
	1.8 g in 1,000 mL
	Glucose 4 g in 100 mL
	40 g in 1,000 mL
	Answer: Potassium, 3 g; sodium, 1.8 g; glucose, 40 g
Question 3	0.45 g in 100 mL
	0.45 g × 5 = 2.25 g in 500 mL
	Answer: 2.25 g
Question 4	Calcium gluconate 10% is equal to 10 g in 100 mL.
	Therefore in a 10 mL ampoule there is 1 g of calcium gluconate.
	But you need 2 g, i.e. 2 ampoules = 2 g or 20 mL calcium gluconate 10%.
	Answer: You need to draw up 20 mL, i.e. 2 ampoules
Question 5	**Answer:** 4.5 mg/mL (multiply by 10)
Question 6	**Answer:** 5 mg/mL (multiply by 10)
Question 7	**Answer:** Potassium, 2 mg/mL; sodium, 1.8 mg/mL; glucose, 40 mg/mL (multiply by 10)
Question 8	0.25% (divide by 10)
Question 9	50% (divide by 10)
Question 10	This last one is slightly different in that the strength is given in micrograms. So first you have to convert this to milligrams by dividing by 1,000:

$$\frac{500}{1,000} = 0.5 \, mg$$

Then divide by 10 as usual.

Answer: 0.05%

Question 11   1 in 200,000 means: 1 g in 200,000 mL.
However, you have a 20 mL vial.
First convert 1 g to milligrams:

$$1,000 \text{ mg in } 200,000 \text{ mL}$$

Next work out how many milligrams in 1 mL:

$$\frac{1,000}{200,000} \text{ mg in } 1 \text{ mL (using the 'ONE unit' rule)}$$

Now work out how much is in the 20 mL vial:

$$\frac{1,000}{200,000} \times 20 = 0.1 \text{ mg in } 20 \text{ mL}$$

Answer: is 0.1 mg or 100 mcg adrenaline/ epinephrine

Question 12   0.7 ppm means 0.7 g in 1,000,000 mL, or 0.7 mg in 1 litre.

$$0.7 \text{ mg} = 700 \text{ micrograms}$$

Answer: 700 micrograms per litre

Chapter 6 Dosage calculations

Question 1   **Answer:** Two 250 mg tablets

Question 2   You need alfacalcidol 1 micrograms. First, ensure units are the same – convert the amount needed to nanograms:

$$1 \text{ micrograms} = 1,000 \text{ nanograms}$$

Each capsule contains 250 nanograms, so how many capsules contain 1,000 nanograms?
   Divide the dose needed (1,000 nanograms) by the strength of the capsule (250 nanograms). Thus:

$$\frac{1,000}{250} = 4$$

Answer: Four 250 nanogram capsules

Question 3

$$\text{Dose} = 1.5 \text{ mg/kg}$$
$$\text{Patient's weight} = 73 \text{ kg}$$

Therefore, to calculate the total dose required, multiply:

$$1.5 \times 73 = 109.5$$

Thus you will need 109.5 mg (rounding up = 110 mg).
Answer: 110 mg

Question 4   Answer: 720 mg

Question 5   Answer: 97 mg

Question 6   Answer: 186 mg

Question 7   Answer: (i) 21,600 mcg; (ii) 21.6 mg (22 mg)

Question 8   Answer: 325 mcg/min

Question 9

$$\text{Dose} = 175 \text{ units/kg}$$
$$\text{Patient weight} = 68 \text{ kg}$$
$$\text{Therefore dose required} = 175 \times 68 = 11{,}900 \text{ units}$$

For a dose of 11,900 units, you will need a 0.7 mL (14,000 units) pre-filled syringe.

Volume to be given: you have 14,000 units in 0.7 mL which is equivalent to:

$$1 \text{ unit in } \frac{0.7}{14{,}000} \text{ mL}$$

Therefore for 11,900 units, you will need:

$$\frac{0.7}{14{,}000} \times 11{,}900 = 0.595 \text{ mL or 0.6 mL (rounding up)}$$

In reality, you would round up the dose to 12,000 units and give 0.6 mL as calibrated on the 0.7mL syringe.

Answer: 12,000 units, i.e give 0.6 mL from a 0.7mL syringe

Question 10

$$\text{Dose} = 1.5 \text{ mg/kg}$$
$$\text{Patient weight} = 59 \text{ kg}$$
$$\text{Therefore dose required} = 1.5 \times 59 = 88.5 \text{ mg}$$

For a dose of 88.5 mg, you will need a 1 mL syringe (10,000 units, 100 mg).

Volume to be given: you have 100 mg in 1 mL, which is equivalent to:

$$1 \text{ mg in } \frac{1}{100} \text{ mL}$$

Therefore for 88.5 mg, you will need:

$$\frac{1}{100} \times 88.5 = 0.885 \text{ mL or 0.9 mL (rounding up)}$$

In reality, you would round up the dose to 90 mg and give 0.9 mL as calibrated on the syringe.

Answer: 90 mg, 0.9 mL syringe

Question 11 Using the formula:

$$BSA\,(m^2) = \sqrt{\frac{height\,(cm)\,\times\,weight\,(kg)}{3,600}}$$

Height = 108 cm, weight = 20 kg; substitute the figures in the formula:

$$BSA = \sqrt{\frac{108 \times 20}{3,600}}$$

$$= \sqrt{\frac{2,160}{3,600}}$$

$$= \sqrt{0.6}$$

$$= 0.77\,m^2$$

Answer: $0.77\,m^2$

Question 12 Using the formula:

$$BSA\,(m^2) = \sqrt{\frac{height\,(cm)\,\times\,weight\,(kg)}{3,600}}$$

Height = 180 cm, weight = 96 kg; substitute the figures in the formula:

$$BSA = \sqrt{\frac{180 \times 96}{3,600}}$$

$$= \sqrt{\frac{17,280}{3,600}}$$

$$= \sqrt{4.8}$$

$$= 2.19\,m^2$$

Answer: $2.19\,m^2$

Question 13 You have erythromycin suspension 250 mg/5 mL.

$$1\text{ mg of suspension} = \frac{5}{250}\text{ mL (using the 'ONE unit' rule)}$$

Dose = 1,000 mg (1 g), which will equal:

$$1,000 \times \frac{5}{250} = 20\,mL$$

Answer: 20 mL of erythromycin suspension 250 mg/5 mL

Question 14 You have digoxin liquid 50 micrograms/mL.

$$1\text{ microgram of liquid} = \frac{1}{50}\text{ mL (using the 'ONE unit' rule)}$$

Dose = 62.5 micrograms, which will equal:

$$62.5 \times \frac{1}{50} = 1.25 \, mL$$

Answer: 1.25 mL of digoxin liquid 50 micrograms/mL

Question 15   You have Oramorph® liquid 100 mg/5 mL.

1 mg of liquid $= \dfrac{5}{100}$ mL (using the 'ONE unit' rule)

Dose = 60 mg which will equal:

$$60 \times \frac{5}{100} = 3 \, mL$$

Answer: 3 mL of Oramorph® liquid 100 mg/5 mL

Question 16   You have pethidine injection 100 mg/2 mL.

1 mg of injection $= \dfrac{2}{100}$ mL (using the 'ONE unit' rule)

Dose = 75 mg, which will equal:

$$75 \times \frac{2}{100} = 1.5 \, mL$$

Answer: 1.5 mL of pethidine injection 100 mg/2 mL

Question 17

$$dose = 2 \, mg/kg$$
$$weight = 23 \, kg$$
$$dose \; required = dose \times weight = 2 \times 23 = 46 \, mg$$

You have ranitidine liquid 150 mg in 10 mL.
Therefore for 46 mg you will need:

$$\frac{10}{150} \times 46 = 3.07 \, mL = 3 \, mL \; (rounded \; down)$$

Sometimes it is necessary to 'adjust' the dose like this for ease of calculation and administration, as long as the 'adjustment' is not too much as to make a large difference in the dose.

Answer: 3 mL of ranitidine liquid 150 mg in 10 mL

Question 18

$$Total \; amount \; required = 18.45 \times 4 = 73.8 \, mg = weight \times dose$$

You have trimethoprim suspension 50 mg/5 mL.

1 mg $= \dfrac{5}{50}$ mL of suspension (using the 'ONE unit' rule)

Dose = 73.8 mg, which will equal:

$$73.8 \times \frac{5}{50} = 7.4 \text{ mL (rounded up)}$$

Answer: 7.4 mL of trimethoprim suspension 50 mg/5 mL

Question 19 The prescribed dose is 2.5 mg/kg daily in two divided doses. and the patient weighs 68 kg, so the total daily dose (TDD) is:

$$TDD = 2.5 \times 68 = 170 \text{ mg}$$

This has to be given in two divided doses, so:

$$\text{each dose} = \frac{170}{2} = 85 \text{ mg}$$

The capsules are available in 10 mg, 25 mg, 50 mg and 100 mg strengths, so you will need to give:

$$
\begin{array}{r}
1 \times 50 \text{ mg} \\
1 \times 25 \text{ mg} \\
1 \times \underline{10 \text{ mg}} + \\
\hline
85 \text{ mg}
\end{array}
$$

Answer: One 10 mg capsule, one 25 mg capsule and one 50 mg capsule

Question 20   Dose required = $76 \times 5 = 380$ mg

Two 250 mg vials acidovir (acyclovir)

Question 21

Dose required for the patient = $50 \times 0.5 = 25$ mg/hour

Therefore for 12 hours, you will need:

$$25 \times 12 = 300 \text{ mg}$$

You have 250 mg in 10 mL. Therefore 1 mg would equal

$$1 \text{ mg} = \frac{10}{250} \text{ mL (using the 'ONE unit' rule).}$$

Thus: $300 \text{ mg} = 1 \text{ mg} = \dfrac{10}{250} \times 300 = 12 \text{ mL}$

Answer: 12 mL

Question 22

i) Total daily dose = weight $\times$ dose = $120 \times 68 = 8,160$ mg

However, it is to be given in four divided doses. Therefore, for each dose, you will need:

$$\frac{8,160}{4} = 2,040 \text{ mg}$$

You have co-trimoxazole ampoules containing 96 mg/mL. Thus:

$$1 \text{ mg} = \frac{1}{96} \text{ mL}$$

Therefore for 2,040 mg you will need:

$$\frac{1}{96} \times 2,040 = 21.25 \text{ mL}$$

Answer: 21.25 mL per dose

ii) Each ampoule contains 5 mL. To work out how many ampoules are needed, divide the total volume required by the volume of each ampoule, i.e.

$$\frac{21.25}{5} = 4.25$$

Therefore you will need five ampoules (25 mL) for each dose, drawing up 21.25 mL and discarding the remainder.

Answer: 5 ampoules per dose

iii) Since it is to be given in four divided doses; to calculate how many ampoules are needed for 1 day, multiply the amount for each dose by 4, i.e.

$$5 \times 4 = 20 \text{ ampoules}$$

Answer: 20 ampoules per 24 hours

iv) 1 ampoule must be diluted to 125 mL, thus for 4.25 ampoules, you will need:

$$4.25 \times 125 = 531.25 \text{ mL}$$

Therefore give in 1 litre sodium chloride infusion 0.9%.

Answer: 1 litre sodium chloride 0.9%

Question 23

i) Displacement volume = 0.8 mL per 1 g vial

Work out how much Water for Injections you need to add to make a final volume of 10 mL:

$$10 \text{ mL} - 0.8 \text{ mL} = 9.2 \text{ mL}$$

Therefore you need to add 9.2 mL Water for Injection to each vial.

ii) The next step is to calculate the volume for 350 mg.

Now you have a final concentration of 100 mg/mL (1 g or 1,000 mg per 10 mL):

$$100 \, \text{mg in } 1 \, \text{mL}$$

$$350 \, \text{mg} = \left(\frac{1}{100} \times 350 \right) \text{mL} = 3.5 \, \text{mL (using the 'ONE unit' rule)}$$

Answer: You need to draw up a dose of 3.5 mL (350 mg).

Question 24

i) Displacement value = 0.5 mL for 1 g

Work out how much Water for Injections you need to add to make a final volume of 4 mL:

$$4 \, \text{mL} - 0.5 \, \text{mL} = 3.5 \, \text{mL}$$

Therefore you need to add 3.5 mL Water for Injections to each vial.

ii) The next step is to calculate the dose:

Now you have a final concentration of 250 mg/mL (1 g or 1,000 mg per 4 mL).

$$\text{Total daily dose} = \text{weight} \times \text{dose} = 18 \times 150 = 2,700 \, \text{mg}$$

$$\text{Each dose} = \frac{2,700}{4} = 675 \, \text{mg}$$

You have 250 mg in 1 mL:

$$675 \, \text{mg} = \left(\frac{1}{250} \times 675 \right) \text{mL} = 2.7 \, \text{mL (using the 'ONE unit' rule)}$$

Answer: For each dose you need to draw up 2.7 mL (675 mg).

Question 25

i) Displacement value = 0.2 mL for 250 mg

Work out how much Water for Injections you need to add to make a final volume of 5 mL:

$$5 \, \text{mL} - 0.2 \, \text{mL} = 4.8 \, \text{mL}$$

Therefore you need to add 4.8 mL water for injection to each vial.

ii) The next step is to calculate the dose:

Now you have a final concentration of 50 mg/mL (250 mg per 5 mL).

$$\text{Dose} = \text{weight} \times \text{dose} = 19.6 \times 12.5 = 245 \, \text{mg}$$

You have 50 mg in 1 mL.

$$245 \, \text{mg} = \frac{1}{50} \times 245 = 4.9 \, \text{mL (using the 'ONE unit' rule)}$$

Answer: For each dose you need to draw up 4.9 mL (245 mg).

Chapter 7 Moles and millimoles

Question 1   One millimole of sodium chloride will give one millimole of sodium.

So the amount (in milligrams) for one millimole of sodium chloride will give one millimole of sodium.

So 58.5 mg (one millimole) of sodium chloride will give one millimole of sodium.

Thus it follows:

1 mg of sodium chloride will give $\dfrac{1}{58.5}$ millimoles of sodium.

Now work out the total amount of sodium chloride in a 500 mL infusion.

You have 27 mg/mL sodium chloride, thus in 500 mL:

$$27 \times 500 = 13{,}500\,mg$$

Next work out the number of millimoles for the infusion:

1 mg will give $\dfrac{1}{58.5}$ millimoles.

13,500 mg will give $\dfrac{1}{58.5} \times 13{,}500 = 230.77\ (231)$ mmol.

Answer: There are 231 mmol (approx.) of sodium in a 500 mL infusion containing sodium chloride 27 mg/mL.

If using the formula:

$$\text{total millimoles} = \frac{\text{mg/mL}}{\text{mg of substance containing 1 mmol}} \times \text{volume (mL)}$$

In this case:

$$\text{mg/mL} = 27$$
$$\text{mg of substance containing 1 mmol} = 58.5$$
$$\text{volume (in mL)} = 500$$

Substituting the numbers in the formula:

$$\frac{27}{58.5} \times 500 = 230.8\ (231)\ \text{mmol.}$$

Answer: There are 231 mmol (approx.) of sodium in a 500 mL infusion containing sodium chloride 27 mg/mL.

Question 2   51.28 mmol (51 mmol, approx.) of sodium

Question 3 Sodium   76.9 mmol (77 mmol, approx.)
           Potassium   20.1 mmol (20 mmol, approx.)
           Chloride   97.0 mmol (97 mmol, approx.)

One millimole of potassium chloride gives one millimole of potassium and **one** millimole of chloride.

One millimole of sodium chloride gives one millimole of sodium and **one** millimole of chloride.

Thus to find the total amount of chloride, add the amount for the sodium and potassium together.

Question 4 277.8 mmol (278 mmol, approx.) of glucose

Question 5 In this question, ignore the glucose since it contains no sodium; simply consider the infusion as sodium chloride 0.18%.

One millimole of sodium chloride will give one millimole of sodium.

So the amount (in milligrams) for one millimole of sodium chloride will give one millimole of sodium.

You are given the molecular mass of sodium chloride = 58.5.

So 58.5 mg (one millimole) of sodium chloride will give one millimole of sodium.

Now work out the number of millimoles for 1 mg of sodium chloride:

58.5 mg sodium chloride will give 1 millimole of sodium.

1 mg sodium chloride will give $\dfrac{1}{58.5}$ millimoles of sodium.

Next, calculate the total amount of sodium chloride present:

$$0.18\% = 0.18\,g \text{ or } 180\,mg \text{ per } 100\,mL$$

Therefore in 1 litre:

$$180 \times 10 = 1{,}800\,mg \text{ sodium chloride}$$

Now calculate the number of millimoles in 1,800 mg sodium chloride:

$$1{,}800\,mg = \frac{1}{58.5} \times 1{,}800 = 30.8\,(31)\ mmol$$

Answer: 1 litre of glucose 4% and sodium chloride 0.18% infusion contains 31 mmol of sodium (approx.).

If using the formula:

$$\text{mmol} = \frac{\text{percentage strength (\% w/v)}}{\text{mg of substance conntaining 1 mmol}} \times 10 \times \text{volume (mL)}$$

In this case:

percentage strength (% w/v) = 0.18
mg of substance containing 1 mmol = 58.5
volume (mL) = 1,000

Substituting the numbers into the formula:

$$\frac{0.18}{58.5} \times 10 \times 1{,}000 = 30.8 \, (31) \, \text{mmol of sodium}$$

Answer: 1 litre of glucose 4% and sodium chloride 0.18% infusion contains 31 mmol of sodium (approx.).

Question 6   In this case one millimole of calcium chloride will give one millimole of calcium and **two** millimoles of chloride.

So the amount (in milligrams) for one millimole of calcium chloride will give one millimole of calcium and two millimoles of chloride.

You are given the molecular mass of calcium chloride = 147.

So 147 mg (one millimole) of calcium chloride will give one millimole of calcium and two millimoles of chloride.

Now calculate how much calcium chloride in the 10 mL ampoule containing calcium chloride 10%.

$$10\% = 10 \, \text{g in 100 mL,}$$
$$\text{therefore: } \frac{10}{10} \, \text{g} = 1 \, \text{g or 1,000 mg in 10 mL}$$

Calcium: 147 mg of calcium chloride contains one millimole of calcium.

Therefore 1 mg calcium chloride contains $\frac{1}{147}$ mmol of calcium.

However, you have 1,000 mg of calcium chloride. Thus:

$$1{,}000 \, \text{mg} = \frac{1}{147} \times 1{,}000 = 6.8 \, \text{mmol (7 mmol, approx.) calcium}$$

Chloride: 147 mg of calcium chloride contains **two** millimoles of chloride

Therefore 1 mg calcium chloride is equal to $\frac{2}{147}$ mmol of chloride.

However, you have 1,000 mg of calcium chloride. Thus:

$$1,000\,mg = \frac{2}{147} \times 1,000 = 13.6\,mmol\ (14\,mmol,\ approx.)\ chloride$$

Answer: There are approximately 7 millimoles of calcium and 14 millimoles of chloride in a 10 mL ampoule of calcium chloride 10%.

If using the formula:

$$mmol = \frac{percentage\ strength\ (\%\ w/v)}{mg\ of\ substance\ conntaining\ 1\ mmol} \times 10 \times volume\ (mL)$$

For **calcium**:

$$percentage\ strength\ (\%\ w/v) = 10$$
$$mg\ of\ substance\ containing\ 1\ mmol = 147$$
$$volume\ (mL) = 10$$

Substituting the numbers into the formula:

$$\frac{10}{147} \times 10 \times 10 = 6.8\,mmol\ (7\,mmol,\ approx.)\ calcium$$

For **chloride**:

$$percentage\ strength\ (\%\ w/v) = 10$$
$$mg\ of\ substance\ containing\ 1\ mmol = 73.5$$
$$volume = 10$$

N.B. mg of substance containing ONE mmol = 73.5:

This is because 2 mmol of chloride = 147 mg, thus

$$1\ mmol\ chloride = \frac{147}{2} = 73.5\,mg$$

Substituting the numbers into the formula:

$$\frac{10}{73.5} \times 10 \times 10 = 13.6\,mmol\ (14\,mmol,\ approx.)\ chloride$$

Answer: There are approximaetly 7 millimoles of calcium and 14 millimoles of chloride in a 10 mL ampoule of calcium chloride 10%.

Question 7   2.23 mmol (2 mmol, approx.) calcium

Question 8   200 mmol sodium

Question 9   First, write down the weight of one mole:

$$1 \text{ mole of sodium bicarbonate} = 84\text{ g}$$

Next calculate the number of moles for 1 g (using the 'ONE unit' rule):

$$1 \text{ g would equal } \frac{1}{84} \text{ mole}$$

Then calculate the number of moles for 8.4 g:

$$8.4\text{ g} = \frac{1}{84} \times 8.4 = \frac{8.4}{84} = 0.1 \text{ moles}$$

You therefore have 0.1 moles of sodium bicarbonate in 50 mL.
    To convert this to a molar concentration, you need to calculate the equivalent number of moles per litre (1,000 mL).
    You have 0.1 moles in 50 mL, which is equal to:

$$1 \text{ mL} = \frac{0.1}{50} \text{ moles}$$

Therefore for 1,000 mL:

$$\frac{0.1}{50} \times 1,000 = \frac{100}{50} = 2 \text{ moles}$$

Answer: If 8.4 g of sodium bicarbonate is made up to 50 mL, the resulting solution would have a concentration of 2 M.

Alternatively, a formula can be used:

$$\text{concentration (mol/L or M)} = \frac{\text{weight (g)} \times 1,000}{\text{molecular weight} \times \text{final volume (mL)}}$$

In this case:

$$\text{weight (g)} = 8.4$$
$$\text{molecular mass} = 84$$
$$\text{final volume (mL)} = 50$$

Substituting the figures into the formula:

$$\frac{8.4 \times 1,000}{84 \times 50} = 2\text{ M}$$

Answer: If 8.4 g of sodium bicarbonate is made up to 50 mL, the resulting solution would have a concentration of 2 M.

Question 10 First, write down the final concentration needed and what it signifies:

$$0.1 \text{ M} = 0.1 \text{ moles in } 1,000 \text{ mL}$$

Next, work out the number of moles needed for the volume required.

You have 0.1 moles in 1,000 mL.

$$\text{Therefore in } 1 \text{ mL} = \frac{0.1}{1,000} \text{ moles}$$

For 250 mL, you will need:

$$\frac{0.1}{1,000} \times 250 = \frac{0.1}{4} = 0.025 \text{ moles}$$

Now convert moles to grams.

You know that 1 mole sodium citrate is equal to 294 g:

$$1 \text{ mole} = 294 \text{ g}$$

Therefore, 0.025 moles = 294 × 0.025 = 7.35 g

Answer: If 7.35 g of sodium citrate is made up to 250 mL, the resulting solution would have a concentration of 0.1 M.

Alternatively, a formula can be used:

$$\text{weight (g)} = \frac{\text{concentration (mol/L or M)} \times \text{molecular weight} \times \text{final volume (mL)}}{1,000}$$

In this case:

$$\text{desired concentration (mol/L or M)} = 0.1$$
$$\text{molecular mass} = 294$$
$$\text{final volume (mL)} = 250$$

Substituting these figures into the formula:

$$\frac{0.1 \times 294 \times 250}{1,000} = 7.35 \text{ g}$$

Answer: If 7.35 g of sodium citrate is made up to 250 mL, the resulting solution would have a concentration of 0.1 M.

Chapter 8 Infusion rate calculations

Question 1   First convert the volume to a number of drops. To do this, multiply the volume of the infusion by the number of drops per mL for the standard giving set:

$$500 \times 20 = 10{,}000 \text{ drops}$$

Next convert hours to minutes by multiplying the number of hours the infusion is to be given by 60.

$$6 \text{ hours} = 6 \times 60 = 360 \text{ minutes}$$

Write down what you have just calculated, i.e. the total number of drops to be given over how many minutes:

$$10{,}000 \text{ drops over } 360 \text{ minutes}$$

Calculate the number of drops per minute by dividing the number of drops by the number of minutes:

$$\text{drops/min} = \frac{10{,}000}{360} = 27.78 \text{ drops/min}$$

(28 drops/min, approx.)

Answer: To give 500 mL of sodium chloride 0.9% over 6 hours, the rate will have to be 28 drops/min using a standard giving set (20 drops/mL).

If using the formula:

$$\text{drops/min} = \frac{\text{drops/mL of the giving set} \times \text{volume of the infusion}}{\text{number of hours the infusion is to run} \times 60}$$

In this case:

drops/mL of the giving set = 20 drops/mL (SGS)
volume of the infusion (in mL) = 500 mL
number of hours the infusion is to run = 6 hours

Substituting the numbers into the formula:

$$\frac{20 \times 500}{6 \times 60} = 27.78 \text{ drops/min (28 drops/min, approx.)}$$

Answer: To give 500 mL of sodium chloride 0.9% over 6 hours, the rate will have to be 28 drops/min using a standard giving set (20 drops/mL).

Question 2   27.7 drops/min (28 drops/min.) – SGS (20 drops/mL)

Question 3   20.8 drops/min (21 drops/min.) – SGS (15 drops/mL)

Question 4   Dose = 10 mcg/min. The final answer is in terms of hours, so multiply by 60 to convert minutes into hours:

Dose = 10 mcg/min = 10 × 60 = 600 mcg/hour

Convert mcg to mg by dividing by 1,000:

$$\frac{600}{1,000} = 0.6\,mg/hour$$

The next step is to calculate the volume for the dose required. Calculate the volume for 1 mg of drug:

You have: 50 mg in 500 mL.

$$1\,mg = \frac{500}{50} = 10\,mL$$

Thus for the dose of 0.6 mg, the volume is equal to:

0.6 mg = 0.6 × 10 = 6 mL/hour

Answer: The rate required is 6 mL/hour.

As the dose is being given as a total dose (not on a weight basis), the following formula can be used:

$$mL/hour = \frac{volume\ to\ be\ infused \times dose \times 60}{amount\ of\ drug \times 1,000}$$

where:

total volume to be infused = 500 mL
total amount of drug (mg) = 50 mg
dose = 10 mcg/min
60 converts minutes to hours

Substitute the numbers in the formula:

$$\frac{500 \times 10 \times 60}{50 \times 1,000} = 6\,mL/hour$$

Answer: The rate required is 6 mL/hour.

Question 5   Dose = 2 mg/min. The final answer is in terms of hours, so multiply by 60 to convert minutes into hours:

dose = 2 mg/min = 2 × 60 = 120 mg/hour

Calculate the volume for 1 mg of drug.

You have: 0.2% which is 0.2 g in 100 mL; in 500 mL, 0.2 × 5 = 1 g or 1,000 mg:

$$1\,mg = \frac{500}{1,000} = 0.5\,mL$$

Thus for the dose of 120 mg, the volume is equal to:

$$120 \times 0.5 = 60 \, mL$$

Answer: The rate required is 60 mL/hour.

As the dose is being given as a total dose (not on a weight basis), the following formula can be used:

$$mL/hour = \frac{\text{volume to be infused} \times \text{dose} \times 60}{\text{amount of drug}}$$

where:

$$\text{total volume to be infused} = 500 \, mL$$
$$\text{total amount of drug (mg)} = 1,000 \, mg$$
$$\text{dose} = 2 \, mg/min$$
$$60 \text{ converts minutes to hours}$$

Substituting the numbers into the formula:

$$\frac{500 \times 2 \times 60}{1,000} = 60 \, mL/hour$$

Answer: The rate required is 60 mL/hour.

Question 6   First calculate the dose required:

$$\text{Dose required} = \text{patient's weight} \times \text{dose prescribed}$$
$$= 80 \times 3 = 240 \, mcg/min$$

Dose = 240 mcg/min. The final answer is in terms of hours, so multiply by 60 to convert minutes into hours:

$$\text{dose} = 240 \times 60 = 14,400 \, mcg/hour$$

Convert mcg to mg by dividing by 1,000:

$$\frac{14,400}{1,000} = 14.4 \, mg/hour$$

The next step is to calculate the volume for the dose required.
   Calculate the volume for 1 mg of drug.
   You have: 800 mg in 500 mL:

$$1 \, mg = \frac{500}{800} = 0.625 \, mL$$

Thus for the dose of 14.4 mg, the volume is equal to:

$$14.4 \times 0.625 = 9 \, mL$$

Answer: The rate required is 9 mL/hour.

Using the formula:

$$\text{mL/hour} = \frac{\text{volume to be infused} \times \text{dose} \times \text{weight} \times 60}{\text{amount of drug} \times 1,000}$$

In this case:

total volume to be infused = 500 mL

total amount of drug (mg) = 800 mg

dose = 3 mcg/kg/min

patient's weight = 80 kg

Substituting the numbers into the formula:

$$\frac{500 \times 3 \times 80 \times 60}{800 \times 1,000} = \frac{5 \times 3 \times 6}{10} = \frac{90}{10} = 9 \text{ mL/hour}$$

Answer: The rate required is 9 mL/hour.

Question 7   (i) Dose required for the patient = 63 × 0.5 = 31.5 mg/hour

Therefore for 12 hours, you will need 31.5 × 12 = 378 mg. You have 250 mg in 10 mL.

Therefore 1 mg would equal $\dfrac{10}{250}$ mL ('ONE unit' rule):

Thus, the volume for 378 mg is:

$$\frac{10}{250} \times 378 = 15.12 \text{ mL (15 mL rounded down)}$$

Answer: Add 15 mL (378 mg) to a 500 mL infusion bag.

(ii) As the infusion is to run over 12 hours, calculate the hourly rate:

500 mL to be given over 12 hours

$$\frac{500}{12} = 41.67 \text{ mL/hour (41.7 mL/hour rounded up)}$$

Answer: 41.7 mL/hour

Question 8   (i) First calculate the dose required:

$$5 \times 86 = 430 \text{ mg}$$

Next, calculate the volume of the reconstituted vial required:

$$500 \text{ mg} = 20 \text{ mL}$$
$$1 \text{ mg} = \frac{20}{500} \text{ mL}$$

Therefore for 430 mg:

$$430 \text{ mg} = \frac{20}{500} \times 430 = 17.2 \text{ mL (17 mL rounded down)}$$

Answer: Add 17 mL (430 mg) to a 100 mL infusion bag.

(ii) As the infusion is to run over 60 minutes, which is the same as 1 hour, then no further calculation is needed. Set the rate to 100 mL/hour.

Answer: 100 mL/hour

Question 9   Dose = 150 mcg/min. The final answer is in terms of hours, so multiply by 60 to convert minutes into hours:

$$150 \times 60 = 9,000 \text{ mcg/hour}$$

Convert mcg to mg by dividing by 1,000:

$$\frac{9,000}{1,000} = 9 \text{ mg/hour}$$

The next step is to calculate the volume for the dose required.
 Calculate the volume for 1 mg of drug:
 You have: 50 mg in 50 mL:

$$1 \text{ mg} = \frac{50}{50} = 1 \text{ mL}$$

Thus for the dose of 9 mg, the volume is equal to:

$$9 \times 1 = 9 \text{ mL/hour}$$

Answer: The rate required is 9 mL/hour.

As the dose is being given as a total dose (not on a weight basis), the following formula can be used:

$$\text{mL/hour} = \frac{\text{volume to be infused} \times \text{dose} \times 60}{\text{amount of drug}}$$

where:

$$\text{total volume to be infused} = 50 \text{ mL}$$
$$\text{total amount of drug (mg)} = 50 \text{ mg}$$
$$\text{dose} = 150 \text{ mcg/min}$$
$$1,000 \text{ converts mcg to mg}$$
$$60 \text{ converts minutes to hours}$$

Substitute the numbers in the formula:

$$\frac{50 \times 150 \times 60}{50 \times 1,000} = 9 \text{ mL/hour}$$

Answer: The rate required is 9 mL/hour.

Question 10   First calculate the dose required:

dose required = patient's weight × dose prescribed
= 75 × 6 = 450 mcg/min

Dose = 450 mcg/min. The final answer is in terms of hours, so multiply by 60 to convert minutes into hours:

450 × 60 = 27,000 mcg/hour

Convert mcg to mg by dividing by 1,000:

$$\frac{27,000}{1,000} = 27 \, \text{mg/hour}$$

The next step is to calculate the volume for the dose required.
Calculate the volume for 1 mg of drug:
You have: 250 mg in 50 mL.

$$\frac{50}{250} = 0.2 \, \text{mL}$$

Thus for the dose of 27 mg, the volume required is:

27 × 0.2 = 5.4 mL

Answer: The rate required is 5.4 mL/hour.
Alternatively, using the formula:

$$\text{mL/hour} = \frac{\text{volume to be infused} \times \text{dose} \times \text{weight} \times 60}{\text{amount of drug} \times 1,000}$$

In this case:

total volume to be infused = 50 mL
total amount of drug (mg) = 250 mg
dose = 6 mcg/kg/min
patient's weight = 75 kg
60 converts minutes to hours
1,000 converts mcg to mg

Substituting the numbers into the formula:

$$\frac{50 \times 6 \times 75 \times 60}{250 \times 1,000} = 5.4 \, \text{mL/hour}$$

Answer: The rate required is 5.4 mL/hour.

Question 11   (i) You need a final concentration of 5 mg/mL which is the same as:

$$1 \, \text{mg} = \frac{1}{5} \, \text{mL}$$

A dose of 1 g = 1,000 mg would need:

$$\frac{1}{5} \times 1,000 = 200\,mL$$

Nearest commercial bag size is 250 mL.

Answer: 250 mL

(ii) Maximum rate is 10 mg/minute, i.e. for every minute give 10 mg vancomycin.

So 1 mg needs to be given over at least $\frac{1}{10}$ minutes.
For a dose of 1 g or 1,000 mg:

$$\frac{1}{10} \times 1,000 = 100 \text{ minutes}$$

Answer: To be given over at least 100 minutes.

(iii) We need to give 250 mL fluid over 100 minutes.

As the pump needs to be set at a rate per hour, we need to calculate the volume to be given over 60 minutes:

$$1 \text{ minute} = \frac{250}{100}\,mL$$

So over 60 minutes: $\frac{250}{100} \times 60 = 150\,mL/hour$

Answer: 150 mL/hour

Question 12 (i) First calculate the dose required:

$$\text{dose required} = \text{patient's weight} \times \text{dose prescribed}$$
$$= 73 \times 5 = 365\,mcg/min$$

Answer: 365 mcg/min

(ii) You have 250 mg in 500 mL.

$$\frac{250}{500} = 0.5\,mg/mL$$

Answer: 0.5 mg/mL or 500 mcg/mL

(iii) Dose = 365 mcg/min. The final answer is in terms of hours, so multiply by 60 to convert minutes into hours:

$$365 \times 60 = 21,900\,mcg/hour$$

Convert mcg to mg by dividing by 1,000:

$$\frac{21,900}{1,000} = 21.9\,mg/hour$$

The next step is to calculate the volume for the dose required.
Calculate the volume for 1 mg of drug.

You have 250 mg in 500 mL:

$$1\,mg = \frac{250}{500} = 2\,mL$$

Thus for the dose of 21.9 mg, the volume is equal to:

$$21.9 \times 2 = 43.8\,mL$$

Answer: The rate required is 43.8 mL/hour.

Question 13 (i) The rate = 2 mg/hour; convert mg to mL.
You have 50 mg in 500 mL:

$$\text{Therefore } 1\,mg = \frac{500}{50} = 10\,mL$$
$$\text{Thus } 2\,mg/hour = 10 \times 2 = 20\,mL/hour$$

Answer: The rate is 20 mL/hour.

(ii) The new rate of 5 mg/hour

$$10 \times 5 = 50\ mL/hour$$

Answer: The rate is now 50 mL/hour.

Question 14 You have 200 mg of dopamine in 50 mL.
First calculate the amount in 1 mL:

You have 200 mg in 50 mL;

$$1\,mL = \frac{200}{50}\,mg = 4\,mg \text{ (using the 'ONE unit' rule)}$$

The rate at which the pump is running is 4 mL/hour; in mg/hour this is:

$$4 \times 4 = 16\,mg/hour$$

Convert milligrams to micrograms by multiplying by 1,000:

$$16 \times 1,000 = 16,000\,mcg/hour$$

Now calculate the rate per minute by dividing by 60 (converts hours to minutes):

$$\frac{16,000}{60} = 266.67\,mcg/min$$

The final step in the calculation is to work out the rate according to the patient's weight (89 kg):

$$\frac{266.67}{89} = 2.996\,mcg/kg/min \approx 3\,mcg/kg/min$$

Answer: The dose is correct: no adjustment is necessary.

Using the formula:

$$\text{mcg/kg/min} = \frac{\text{rate (mL/hour)} \times \text{amount of drug} \times 1,000}{\text{weight (kg)} \times \text{volume (mL)} \times 60}$$

where, in this case:

$$\text{rate} = 4\,\text{mL/hour}$$
$$\text{amount of drug (mg)} = 200\,\text{mg}$$
$$\text{weight (kg)} = 89\,\text{kg}$$
$$\text{volume (mL)} = 50\,\text{mL}$$
$$60 \text{ converts minutes to hours}$$
$$1,000 \text{ converts mg to mcg}$$

Substituting the numbers into the formula:

$$\frac{4 \times 200 \times 1,000}{89 \times 50 \times 60} = 2.99\,\text{mcg/kg/min} \approx 3\,\text{mcg/kg/min}$$

Answer: The dose is correct: no adjustment is necessary.

Question 15   You have 250 mg of dobutamine in 50 mL.
First calculate the amount in 1 mL:

You have 250 mg in 50 mL:

$$1\,\text{mL} = \frac{250}{50}\,\text{mg} = 5\,\text{mg (using the 'ONE unit' rule)}$$

The rate at which the pump is running is 5.4 mL/hour, therefore in mg/hour this is:

$$5.4\,\text{mL/hour} = 5.4 \times 5 = 27\,\text{mg/hour}$$

Convert milligrams to micrograms by multiplying by 1,000:

$$27 \times 1,000 = 27,000\,\text{mcg/hour}$$

Now calculate the rate per minute by dividing by 60 (converts hours to minutes):

$$\frac{27,000}{60} = 450\,\text{mcg/min}$$

Next work out the rate according to the patient's weight (64 kg):

$$\frac{450}{64} = 7.03\,\text{mcg/kg/min}$$

Answer: 7.03 mcg/kg/min (7 mcg/kg/min, rounded down); the dose being delivered by the pump set at a rate of 5.4 mL/hour is too high, so inform the doctor and adjust the rate of the pump.

Using the formula:

$$\text{mcg/kg/min} = \frac{\text{rate (mL/hour)} \times \text{amount of drug} \times 1,000}{\text{weight (kg)} \times \text{volume (mL)} \times 60}$$

where in this case:

rate $= 5.4$ mL/hour

amount of drug (mg) $= 250$ mg

weight (kg) $= 64$ kg

volume (mL) $= 50$ mL

60 converts minutes to hours

1,000 converts mg to mcg

Substitute the numbers in the formula:

$$\frac{5.4 \times 250 \times 1,000}{64 \times 50 \times 60} = 7.03 \text{ mcg/kg/min (7 mcg/kg/min)}$$

Answer: 7.03 mcg/kg/min (7 mcg/kg/min, rounded down); the dose being delivered by the pump set at a rate of 5.4 mL/hour is too high, so inform the doctor and adjust the rate of the pump.

CHANGING THE RATE OF THE PUMP

In this case, the calculation is done the other way round – starting at the dose.

First calculate the dose required:

dose required $=$ patient's weight $\times$ dose prescribed

$= 64 \times 6 = 384$ mcg/min

The final answer is in terms of hours, so multiply by 60 to convert minutes into hours:

$$384 \times 60 = 23,040 \text{ mcg/hour}$$

Convert mcg to mg by dividing by 1,000:

$$\frac{23.040}{1,000} = 23.04 \text{ mg/hour}$$

The next step is to calculate the volume for the dose required.

Calculate the volume for 1 mg of drug.

You have: 250 mg in 50 mL

$$1 \text{ mg} = \frac{50}{250} = 0.2 \text{ mL}$$

Thus for the dose of 23.04 mg, the volume is equal to:

$$23.04 \times 0.2 = 4.608 \text{ mL/hour}$$

Answer: The pump should have been set at 4.6 mL/hour. A formula can be used:

$$\text{mL/hour} = \frac{\text{volume to be infused} \times \text{dose} \times \text{weight} \times 60}{\text{amount of drug} \times 1,000}$$

In this case:

$$\text{total volume to be infused} = 50\,\text{mL}$$
$$\text{total amount of drug (mg)} = 250\,\text{mg}$$
$$\text{dose} = 6\,\text{mcg/kg/min}$$
$$\text{patient's weight} = 64\,\text{kg}$$
$$60\,\text{converts minutes to hours}$$
$$1,000\,\text{converts mcg to mg}$$

Substituting the numbers into the formula:

$$\frac{50 \times 6 \times 64 \times 60}{250 \times 1,000} = 4.608\,\text{mL/hour (4.6 mL/hour, approx.)}$$

Answer: The rate at which the pump should have been set is 4.6 mL/hour.

Question 16 You have 50 mg of dopexamine in 50 mL.
First calculate the amount in 1 mL:

You have 50 mg in 50 mL:

$$1\,\text{mL} = \frac{50}{50}\,\text{mg} = 1\,\text{mg (using the 'ONE unit' rule)}$$

The rate at which the pump is running is 28 mL/hour, therefore in mg/hour this is:

$$28 \times 1 = 28\,\text{mg/hour}$$

Convert milligrams to micrograms by multiplying by 1,000:

$$28 \times 1,000 = 28,000\,\text{mcg/hour}$$

Now calculate the rate per minute by dividing by 60 (converts hours to minutes):

$$\frac{28,000}{60} = 466.67\,\text{mcg/min}$$

The final step in the calculation is to work out the rate according to the patient's weight (78 kg):

$$\frac{466.67}{78} = 5.98\,\text{mcg/kg/min} \approx 6\,\text{mcg/kg/min rounded up}$$

Answer: The dose is correct: no adjustment is necessary.
Using the formula:

$$mcg/kg/min = \frac{rate\ (mL/hour) \times amount\ of\ drug \times 1,000}{weight\ (kg) \times volume\ (mL) \times 60}$$

where in this case:

$$rate = 28\,mL/hour$$
$$amount\ of\ drug\ (mg) = 50\,mg$$
$$weight\ (kg) = 78\,kg$$
$$volume\ (mL) = 50\,mL$$
$$60\ converts\ minutes\ to\ hours$$
$$1,000\ converts\ mg\ to\ mcg$$

Substituting the numbers into the formula:

$$\frac{28 \times 50 \times 1,000}{78 \times 50 \times 60} = 5.98\,mcg/kg/min \approx 6\,mcg/kg/min\ \text{'rounded up'}$$

Answer: The dose is correct: no adjustment is necessary.

Question 17   First, convert the volume to drops by multiplying the volume of the infusion by the number of drops/mL for the giving set:

$$500 \times 20 = 10,000\ drops$$

Next, calculate how many minutes it will take for 1 drop:

$$42\ drops\ per\ minute$$
$$1\ drop\ will\ take\ \frac{1}{42}\ min$$

Calculate how many minutes it will take to infuse the total number of drops:

$$10,000\ drops\ will\ take\ \frac{1}{42} \times 10,000 = 238\,min$$

Convert minutes to hours by dividing by 60:

$$238\,min = \frac{238}{60} = 3.97\ hours$$

$$3.97\ hours = 3\ hours\ 58\ minutes\ (approx.\ 4\ hours)$$

Answer: An infusion of 500 mL of sodium chloride 0.9% at a rate of 42 drops/min will take approximately 4 hours to run.

Using the formula:

$$\text{number of hours the infusion is to run} =$$

$$\frac{\text{volume of the infusion}}{\text{rate (drops/min)} \times 60} \times \text{drip rate of giving set}$$

where, in this case:

$$\text{volume of the infusion} = 500\,\text{mL}$$
$$\text{rate (drops/min)} = 42\,\text{drops/min}$$
$$\text{drip rate of giving set} = 20\,\text{drops/mL}$$

Substituting the numbers into the formula:

$$\frac{500 \times 20}{42 \times 60} = 3.97\,\text{hours}$$

3.97 hours = 3 hours 58 minutes (approx. 4 hours)

Answer: An infusion of 500 mL of sodium chloride 0.9% at a rate of 42 drops/min will take approximately 4 hours to run.

Question 18 Divide the volume by the rate to give you the time over which the infusion is to run:

$$\text{calculated rate} = 83\,\text{mL/hour}$$
$$\text{volume} = 1{,}000\,\text{mL}$$

$$\frac{1{,}000}{83} = 12.05\,\text{hours (12 hours approximately)}$$

Answer: An infusion of 1 litre of sodium chloride 0.9% at a rate of 83 mL/hour will take 12 hours to run.

Using the formula:

Number of hours the infusion is to run =

where in this case:

$$\text{volume of the infusion} = 1{,}000\,\text{mL}$$
$$\text{rate (mL/hour)} = 83\,\text{mL/hour}$$

Substituting the numbers into the formula:

$$\frac{1{,}000}{83} = 12.05\,\text{hours (12 hours approximately)}$$

Answer: An infusion of 1 litre of sodium chloride 0.9% at a rate of 83 mL/hour will take 12 hours to run.

Question 19 Isosorbide dinitrate 0.05%w/v = 0.05 g in 100 mL.
Convert this to milligrams:

$$0.05\,\text{g} = 50\,\text{mg in 100}\,\text{mL}$$

Next, calculate the volume for 2 mg:

You have 50 mg = 100 mL:

$$1\,mg = \frac{100}{50}\,mL \text{ (using the 'ONE unit' rule)}$$
$$2\,mg = \frac{100}{50} \times 2 = 4\,mL$$

Answer: To deliver a dose of 2 mg/hour the pump should be set at a rate of infusion of 4 mL/hour.

Question 20   Flucloxacillin: each 500 mg vial contains 1.13 mmol of sodium.
Total daily dose of flucloxacillin is 4 g.

Convert to milligrams as the vial strength is in milligrams (500 mg):

$$4\,g = 4{,}000\,mg$$

Calculate the number of vials used per day by dividing the total daily dose by the vial strength, i.e.:

$$\frac{4{,}000}{500} = 8 \text{ vials}$$

Total sodium content from the flucloxacillin:

$$8 \times 1.13 = 9.04\,mmol$$

Total sodium content from the sodium chloride 0.9% infusion:
1 litre (1,000 mL) contains 154 mmol.

Total daily fluid needed for administration = 4 × 100 mL.
(Each 1 g is given in 100 mL and you are giving 4 doses.)
If 1,000 mL contains 154 mmol of sodium:

$$1\,mL = \frac{154}{1{,}000}\,mmol \text{ of sodium (using the 'ONE unit' rule)}$$

Then 400 mL will contain:

$$\frac{154}{1{,}000} \times 400 = 61.6\,mmol \text{ of sodium}$$

Total amount of sodium:

$$9.04\,mmol + 61.6\,mmol = 70.64\,mmol$$

Answer: The patient is receiving a total of 70.64 (71) mmol of sodium per day.

Chapter 9 Action and administration of drugs

Question 1	0.37 mL
Question 2	0.83 mL
Question 3	0.56 mL
Question 4	0.75 mL
Question 5	1.4 mL
Question 6	1.8 mL
Question 7	2.7 mL
Question 8	3.6 mL
Question 9	6.5 mL
Question 10	7.75 mL

Appendices

1 Body surface area (BSA) estimates
   - Using formulae
   - Using nomograms
2 Weight conversion tables
3 Height conversion tables
4 Calculation of Body Mass Index (BMI)
5 Estimation of renal function
6 Abbreviations used in prescriptions

Appendix I

BODY SURFACE AREA (BSA) ESTIMATES

Many physiological phenomena correlate to body surface area (BSA) and for this reason some drug doses are calculated using body surface area.

Cancer chemotherapy is usually dosed using BSA. BSA has been chosen rather than body weight to calculate chemotheraphy doses for two reasons:

- It provides a more accurate estimation of effect and toxicity.
- It more closely correlates to blood flow to the liver and kidneys, which are the major organs for drug elimination.

Cancer drugs have a lower therapeutic index (the difference between an effective and a toxic dose) than most other drugs, i.e. the difference between an underdose and an overdose is small and the consequences of a toxic dose can be life-threatening. Therefore, cancer chemotherapy needs a precise and reliable method of determining the BSA and thereby the appropriate dose.

Doses for paediatric use can be estimated more accurately using BSA and some drugs, e.g. acyclovir, have doses based on BSA.

Several different formulae and nomograms have been derived for predicting surface area from measurements of height and weight. For accuracy, BSA should be calculated to three significant figures. Slide rules and nomograms are incapable of calculating with this degree of accuracy. In addition, they suffer from error associated with their analogue nature and the formulae on which they are based.

FORMULAE FOR CALCULATING BODY SURFACE AREA

There are many formulae for calculating BSA. The formula derived by Mosteller (1987) combines an accurate BSA calculation with ease of use, and has been validated for use in both children and adults. This formula can be used on a handheld calculator. It is:

$$m^2 = \sqrt{\frac{\text{height (cm)} \times \text{weight (kg)}}{3,600}}$$

For example, you want to know the body surface area of a child whose weight is 16.4 kg and height is 100 cm.

Substitute the figures into the formula:

$$BSA = \sqrt{\frac{100 \times 16.4}{3,600}}$$

$$= \sqrt{\frac{1,640}{3,600}}$$

$$= \sqrt{0.456}$$

$$= 0.675\, m^2$$

First, do the sum in the top line: $100 \times 16.4 = 1,640$.
Next, divide by 3,600 to give 0.456.
Finally, find the square root to give an answer of $0.675\, m^2$.

NOMOGRAMS

In 1916, Du Bois and Du Bois derived a formula to estimate BSA on which many nomograms are based. Although they used measurements of only nine individuals, one of whom was a child, and made certain assumptions in developing the formula, this remains the most popular nomogram for calculating BSA.

However, many investigators have since questioned the accuracy of the Du Bois formula. Haycock *et al.* (1978) reported that the formula underestimates surface area by up to 8% in infants, especially as values fell below $0.7\, m^2$. Nomograms based on the formula derived by Haycock *et al.* are now used in paediatric books, with separate nomograms for infants (Fig. A1.1, overleaf) and for children and adults (Fig. A1.2, overleaf).

Before you can use the nomogram, you have to know the patient's height and weight. Once these have been measured, a straight-line edge (e.g. a ruler) is placed from the patient's height in the left-hand column to their weight in the right-hand column, and where the line intersects the BSA column indicates the body surface area.

> **TIP BOX**
>
> Using a recognized formula is a more accurate way to calculate BSA than using a nomogram. Nomograms should only be used as a rough guide or estimate.

References

GB Haycock, GJ Schwartz, DH Wisotsky. Geometric method for measuring body surface area: a height–weight formula validated in infants, children and adults. *J Pediatr* 1978; **93**: 62–6.

RD Mosteller. Simplified calculation of body-surface area. *N Engl J Med* 1987; **317**: 1098.

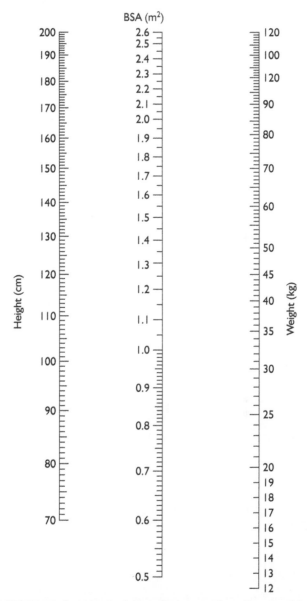

Fig A1.1 Nomogram for estimating body surface area in infants. Reproduced from Documenta Geigy Scientific Tables (1970), with permission from Wiley-Blackwell

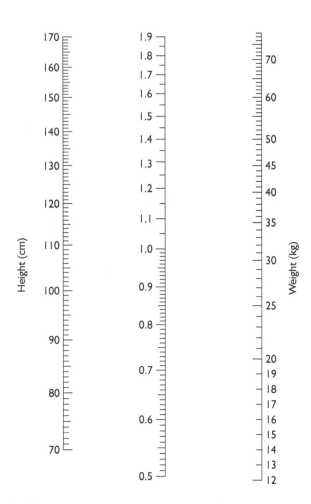

Fig A1.2 Nomogram for estimating body surface area in children and adults. Reproduced from Documenta Geigy Scientific Tables (1970), with permission from Wiley-Blackwell

Appendix 2

WEIGHT CONVERSION TABLES

It may sometimes be necessary to convert stones and pounds to kilograms and vice versa. Patients' weights are usually given in stones and have to be converted to kilograms, especially when working out dosages. A lot of dosages are calculated on a 'weight basis', e.g. mg/kg/day.

The following table shows weight conversions.

| STONES TO KILOGRAMS | | POUNDS TO KILOGRAMS | |
STONES	KILOGRAMS	POUNDS	KILOGRAMS
1	6.4	1	0.5
2	12.7	2	0.9
3	19.1	3	1.4
4	25.4	4	1.8
5	31.8	5	2.3
6	38.1	6	2.7
7	44.5	7	3.2
8	50.8	8	3.6
9	57.2	9	4.1
10	63.5	10	4.5
11	69.9	11	5.0
12	76.2	12	5.4
13	82.6	13	5.9
14	88.9		
15	95.3		
16	101.6		
17	108.0		
18	114.3		
19	120.7		
20	127.0		
21	133.4		

Weights in kg correct to 0.1 kg

Conversion factors
Stones to kilograms ×6.3503
Pounds to kilograms ×0.4536
Kilograms to stones ×0.1575
Kilograms to pounds ×2.2046

WORKED EXAMPLE

Convert 14 stones 4 pounds to kilograms (to the nearest kg).

USING THE CONVERSION TABLE

$$14 \text{ stones} = 88.9 \text{ kg}$$
$$4 \text{ pounds} = \underline{1.8 \text{ kg}} \quad \text{(Add the two together)}$$
$$90.7 \text{ kg}$$

ANSWER: 91 kg (to nearest kg)

USING THE CONVERSION FACTORS

Use the conversion factor: **stones** to **kilograms** (multiply by 6.3503)

$$14 \text{ stones} = 14 \times 6.3503 = 88.9042 \text{ kg}$$

Use the conversion factor: **pounds** to **kilograms** (multiply by 0.4536)

$$4 \text{ pounds} = 4 \times 0.4536 = 1.8144 \text{ kg}$$

14 stones =	88.9042 kg
4 pounds =	1.8144 kg (Add the two together)
	90.7186 kg

ANSWER: 91 kg (to nearest kg)

Appendix 3

HEIGHT CONVERSION TABLES

Sometimes, it may be necessary to convert feet and inches to centimetres and vice versa. Patients' heights are usually given in feet and inches and have to be converted to centimetres. Some dosages are calculated on a 'surface area basis', e.g. mg/m^2, particularly cytotoxic drugs. Formulae to calculate surface area require weight in kilograms and height in centimetres.

The following table shows height conversions.

FEET TO CENTIMETRES		INCHES TO CENTIMETRES	
FEET	**CENTIMETRES**	**INCHES**	**CENTIMETRES**
1	30.5	1	2.5
2	61.0	2	5.1
3	91.4	3	7.6
4	121.9	4	10.2
5	152.4	5	12.7
6	182.9	6	15.2
		7	17.8

Lengths in centimetres correct to 0.1 cm   8   20.3

9   22.9

Conversion factors   10   25.4

Feet to centimetres ×30.48   11   27.9

Inches to centimetres ×2.54

Centimetres to feet ×0.028

Centimetres to inches ×0.3937

WORKED EXAMPLE

Convert 6 feet 2 inches to centimetres (to the nearest cm).

USING THE CONVERSION TABLE

        6 feet =   182.9 cm
        2 inches =   5.1 cm   (Add the two together)
                  ‾‾‾‾‾‾‾‾‾
                   188.0 cm

ANSWER: 188 cm (to nearest cm)

USING THE CONVERSION FACTORS

Use the conversion factor: **feet** to **centimetres** (multiply by 30.48)

$$6 \text{ feet} = 6 \times 30.48 = 182.88 \text{ cm}$$

use the conversion factor: inches to centimetres (multiply by 2.54)

$$2 \text{ inches} = 2 \times 2.54 = 5.08 \text{ cm}$$

$$
\begin{array}{rl}
6 \text{ feet} = & 182.88 \text{ cm} \\
2 \text{ inches} = & \underline{5.08 \text{ cm}} \quad \text{(Add the two together)} \\
& 187.96 \text{ cm}
\end{array}
$$

ANSWER: 188 cm (to nearest cm)

Appendix 4

CALCULATION OF BODY MASS INDEX (BMI)

Body mass index or BMI, based on an individual's height and weight (wt/ht^2), is a helpful indicator of obesity and underweight in adults.

BMI compares well to body fat but cannot be interpreted as a certain percentage of body fat. The relation between fatness and BMI is influenced by age and sex. For example, women are more likely to have a higher percentage of body fat than men for the same BMI. At the same BMI, older people have more body fat than younger adults.

BMI is used to screen and monitor a population to detect risk of health or nutritional disorders. In an individual, other data must be used to determine if a high BMI is associated with increased risk of disease and death for that person. BMI alone is not diagnostic.

A healthy BMI for adults is between 18.5 and 24.9. BMI ranges are based on the effect body weight has on disease and death. A high BMI is predictive of death from cardiovascular disease. Diabetes, cancer, high blood pressure and osteoarthritis are also common consequences of overweight and obesity in adults. Obesity itself is a strong risk factor for premature death.

BMI GUIDELINES

- Underweight: BMI <18.4
- Acceptable: BMI 18.5–24.9
- Overweight: BMI 25–29.9
- Obese: BMI 30–39.9
- Morbidly obese BMI >40

WORKED EXAMPLE

Calculate the BMI for a patient with height 188 cm and weight 91 kg.

$$BMI = \frac{weight\ (kg)}{height \times height\ (m^2)}$$

In this case, height = 1.88 m; 1.88 × 1.88 = 3.53

$$BMI = \frac{91}{3.53} = 25.7 \approx 26$$

From the table, a weight of (91 kg) and a height of (1.88 m) would give a BMI of 26.

Feet			5	5	5	5	5	5	5	5	5	5	5	5	6	6	6	6	6	6	6
Inches			0	1	2	3	4	5	6	7	8	9	10	11	0	1	2	3	4	5	6
Metres			1.52	1.55	1.57	1.6	1.63	1.65	1.68	1.7	1.73	1.75	1.78	1.8	1.83	1.85	1.88	1.91	1.93	1.96	1.98
Stones	Pounds	Kilograms																			
14	4	91	39	38	37	36	34	33	32	31	30	30	29	28	27	27	26	25	24	24	23

Feet			5	5	5	5	5	5	5	5	5	5	5	5	6	6	6	6	6	6	6
Inches			0	1	2	3	4	5	6	7	8	9	10	11	0	1	2	3	4	5	6
Metres			1.52	1.55	1.57	1.6	1.63	1.65	1.68	1.7	1.73	1.75	1.78	1.8	1.83	1.85	1.88	1.91	1.93	1.96	1.98
Stones	Pounds	Kilograms																			
6	0	38	16	16	15	15	14	14	13	13	13	12	12	12	11	11	11	10	10	10	10
6	2	39	17	16	16	15	15	14	14	13	13	13	12	12	12	11	11	11	10	10	10
6	4	40	17	17	16	16	15	15	14	14	13	13	13	12	12	12	11	11	11	10	10
6	6	41	18	17	17	16	15	15	15	14	14	13	13	13	12	12	12	11	11	11	10
6	8	42	18	17	17	16	16	15	15	15	14	14	13	13	13	12	12	12	11	11	11
6	10	43	19	18	17	17	16	16	15	15	14	14	14	13	13	13	12	12	12	11	11
6	12	44	19	18	18	17	17	16	16	15	15	14	14	14	13	13	12	12	12	11	11
7	0	44	19	18	18	17	17	16	16	15	15	14	14	14	13	13	12	12	12	11	11
7	2	45	19	19	18	18	17	17	16	16	15	15	14	14	13	13	13	12	12	12	11

BMI <18.4 = underweight; BMI 18.5–24.9 = acceptable; BMI 25–29.9 = overweight; BMI 30–39.9 = obese; BMI >40 = morbidly obese

Feet	6	6	6	6	6	6	6	5	5	5	5	5	5	5	5	5	5	5	5
Inches	6	5	4	3	2	1	0	11	10	9	8	7	6	5	4	3	2	1	0
Metres	1.98	1.96	1.93	1.91	1.88	1.85	1.83	1.8	1.78	1.75	1.73	1.7	1.68	1.65	1.63	1.6	1.57	1.55	1.52

Stones	Pounds	Kilograms	1.98	1.96	1.93	1.91	1.88	1.85	1.83	1.8	1.78	1.75	1.73	1.7	1.68	1.65	1.63	1.6	1.57	1.55	1.52
7	4	46	12	12	12	13	13	13	14	14	15	15	15	16	16	17	17	18	19	19	20
7	6	47	12	12	13	13	13	14	14	15	15	15	16	16	17	17	18	18	19	20	20
7	8	48	12	12	13	13	14	14	14	15	15	16	16	17	17	18	18	19	19	20	21
7	11	49	12	13	13	13	14	14	15	15	15	16	16	17	17	18	18	19	20	20	21
7	12	50	13	13	13	14	14	15	15	15	16	16	17	17	18	18	19	20	20	21	22
8	0	51	13	13	14	14	14	15	15	16	16	17	17	18	18	19	19	20	21	21	22
8	2	52	13	13	14	14	15	15	16	16	16	17	17	18	18	19	20	20	21	22	23
8	4	53	14	14	14	15	15	15	16	16	17	17	18	18	19	19	20	21	22	22	23
8	6	54	14	14	14	15	15	16	16	17	17	18	18	19	19	20	20	21	22	22	23
8	8	54	14	14	15	15	15	16	16	17	17	18	18	19	19	20	20	21	22	22	23
8	10	55	14	14	15	15	16	16	16	17	18	18	18	19	19	20	21	21	22	23	24
8	12	56	14	15	15	15	16	16	17	17	18	18	19	19	20	21	21	22	23	23	24
9	0	57	15	15	15	16	16	17	17	18	18	19	19	20	20	21	21	22	23	24	25
9	2	58	15	15	16	16	16	17	17	18	18	19	19	20	21	21	22	23	24	24	25
9	4	59	15	15	16	16	17	17	18	18	19	19	20	20	21	22	22	23	24	25	26
9	6	60	15	16	16	16	17	18	18	19	19	20	20	21	21	22	23	23	24	25	26
9	8	61	16	16	16	17	17	18	18	19	19	20	20	21	22	22	23	24	25	25	26
9	10	62	16	16	17	17	18	18	19	19	20	20	21	21	22	23	23	24	25	26	27
9	12	63	16	16	17	17	18	18	19	19	20	21	21	22	22	23	24	25	26	26	27

																			kg	lb	st
16	17	17	18	18	19	19	20	20	21	21	22	23	24	24	25	26	27	28	64	0	10
16	17	17	18	18	19	19	20	20	21	21	22	23	24	24	25	26	27	28	64	2	10
17	17	17	18	18	19	19	20	21	21	22	22	23	24	24	25	26	27	28	65	4	10
17	17	18	18	19	19	20	20	21	22	22	23	23	24	25	26	27	27	29	66	6	10
17	17	18	18	19	20	20	21	21	22	22	23	24	25	25	26	27	28	29	67	8	10
17	18	18	19	19	20	20	21	21	22	23	24	24	25	26	27	28	28	29	68	10	10
18	18	19	19	20	20	21	21	22	23	23	24	24	25	26	27	28	29	30	69	12	10
18	18	19	19	20	20	21	22	22	23	24	24	25	26	26	27	28	29	30	70	0	11
18	18	19	19	20	21	21	22	22	23	24	25	25	26	27	28	29	30	31	71	2	11
18	18	19	20	20	21	21	22	23	24	24	25	26	26	27	28	29	30	31	72	4	11
19	19	19	20	21	21	22	23	23	24	24	25	26	27	27	29	30	30	32	73	6	11
19	19	20	20	21	21	22	23	23	24	25	25	26	27	27	29	30	30	32	73	8	11
19	19	20	20	21	22	22	23	23	24	25	26	26	27	27	29	30	31	32	74	10	11
19	19	20	21	21	22	22	23	24	24	25	26	27	28	28	29	31	31	32	75	12	11
19	19	20	21	22	22	23	23	24	25	26	26	27	28	28	30	31	32	33	76	0	12
20	20	21	21	22	22	23	24	24	25	26	27	27	28	29	30	32	32	33	77	2	12
20	20	21	21	22	23	23	24	25	25	26	27	28	29	29	30	32	32	34	78	4	12
20	20	21	21	22	23	24	24	25	26	27	27	28	29	29	31	32	33	34	79	6	12
20	20	21	22	23	23	24	25	25	26	27	28	28	29	30	31	33	33	35	80	8	12
21	21	21	22	23	24	24	25	26	26	27	28	29	30	30	32	33	34	35	81	10	12
21	21	22	22	23	24	24	25	26	27	28	28	29	30	30	32	33	34	35	82	12	12
21	22	22	23	23	24	25	26	26	27	28	29	29	30	31	32	34	35	36	83	0	13

BMI <18.4 = underweight; BMI 18.5–24.9 = acceptable; BMI 25–29.9 = overweight; BMI 30–39.9 = obese; BMI >40 = morbidly obese

Feet			6	6	6	6	6	6	6	5	5	5	5	5	5	5	5	5	5	5
Inches			6	5	4	3	2	1	0	11	10	9	8	7	6	5	4	3	2	1	0
		Metres	1.98	1.96	1.93	1.91	1.88	1.85	1.83	1.8	1.78	1.75	1.73	1.7	1.68	1.65	1.63	1.6	1.57	1.55	1.52
Stones	Pounds	Kilograms																			
13	2	83	21	22	22	23	23	24	25	26	26	27	28	29	29	30	31	32	34	35	36
13	4	84	21	22	23	23	24	25	25	26	27	27	28	29	30	31	32	33	34	35	36
13	6	85	22	22	23	23	24	25	25	26	27	28	28	29	30	31	32	33	34	35	37
13	8	86	22	22	23	24	24	25	26	27	27	28	29	30	30	32	32	34	35	36	37
13	10	87	22	23	23	24	25	25	26	27	27	28	29	30	31	32	33	34	35	36	38
13	12	88	22	23	24	24	25	26	26	27	28	29	29	30	31	32	33	34	36	37	38
14	0	89	23	23	24	24	25	26	27	27	28	29	30	31	32	33	33	35	36	37	39
14	2	90	23	23	24	25	25	26	27	28	28	29	30	31	32	33	34	35	37	37	39
14	4	91	23	24	24	25	26	27	27	28	29	30	30	32	32	33	34	36	37	38	39
14	6	92	23	24	25	25	26	27	27	28	29	30	31	32	33	34	35	36	37	38	40
14	8	93	24	24	25	25	26	27	28	29	29	30	31	32	33	34	35	36	38	39	40
14	10	93	24	24	25	25	26	27	28	29	29	30	31	32	33	34	35	36	38	39	40
14	12	94	24	24	25	26	26	27	28	29	29	30	31	32	33	35	35	36	38	39	41
15	0	95	24	25	26	26	27	28	29	29	30	31	32	32	34	35	36	37	39	40	41
15	2	96	24	25	26	27	27	28	29	30	30	31	32	33	34	35	36	37	39	40	42
15	4	97	25	25	26	27	27	29	30	30	31	31	32	33	34	36	37	38	39	41	42
15	6	98	25	26	26	27	28	29	29	31	31	32	33	34	35	36	37	38	40	41	42
15	8	99	25	26	27	27	28	29	30	31	31	32	33	34	35	36	37	38	40	41	43
15	10	100	26	26	27	27	28	29	30	31	32	33	33	35	35	37	38	39	41	42	43

26	26	27	28	29	30	30	31	32	33	34	35	36	37	38	39	41	42	44			
26	27	27	28	29	30	30	31	32	33	34	35	36	37	38	40	41	42	44			
27	27	28	28	29	30	31	32	33	34	34	35	36	38	39	40	42	43	45			
28	28	28	28	29	30	31	32	33	34	34	35	36	38	39	40	42	43	45			
29	29	29	29	29	30	31	32	33	34	35	36	37	38	39	41	42	43	45			
30	30	30	30	30	31	31	32	33	34	35	36	37	39	40	41	43	44	46			
30	30	31	31	31	31	32	33	34	35	35	37	38	39	40	41	43	45	46			
31	31	32	32	32	32	33	33	34	35	36	37	38	39	41	42	44	45	47			
32	32	33	33	33	33	34	34	35	36	36	38	39	40	41	43	44	45	47			
33	33	34	34	34	34	35	35	36	36	37	38	39	40	42	43	45	46	48			
34	34	34	34	35	35	35	36	36	37	37	38	39	41	42	43	45	46	48			
35	35	35	35	36	36	37	37	38	38	38	39	40	41	42	44	45	47	48			
36	36	36	36	37	37	38	38	39	39	39	40	41	42	43	44	46	47	49			
37	37	38	38	38	39	39	39	40	40	40	41	42	43	44	45	47	48	50			
38	38	39	39	39	40	40	40	41	41	41	42	43	44	45	46	48	49	51			
39	40	40	40	41	41	41	42	42	43	43	43	44	45	46	47	48	50	52			
41	41	42	42	42	43	43	43	44	44	45	45	45	46	47	48	49	50	52			
42	42	43	43	43	44	45	45	45	46	46	47	47	47	48	48	49	50	52			
44	44	45	45	45	46	46	47	47	48	48	48	48	49	49	50	50	51	51	52	52	
101	102	103	103	104	105	106	107	108	109	110	111	112	112	114	114	115	116	117	118	119	120
12	0	2	4	6	8	10	12	0	2	4	6	8	10	13	0	2	4	6	8	10	12
15	16	16	16	16	16	16	16	17	17	17	17	17	17	17	18	18	18	18	18	18	18

BMI <18.4 = underweight; BMI 18.5–24.9 = acceptable; BMI 25–29.9 = overweight; BMI 30–39.9 = obese; BMI >40 = morbidly obese

Feet	5	5	5	5	5	5	5	5	5	5	5	5	6	6	6	6	6	6	6
Inches	0	1	2	3	4	5	6	7	8	9	10	11	0	1	2	3	4	5	6
Metres	1.52	1.55	1.57	1.6	1.63	1.65	1.68	1.7	1.73	1.75	1.78	1.8	1.83	1.85	1.88	1.91	1.93	1.96	1.98
Stones / Pounds / Kilograms																			
19 / 0 / 121	52	50	49	47	46	44	43	42	40	40	38	37	36	35	34	33	32	31	31
19 / 2 / 122	53	51	49	48	46	45	43	42	41	40	39	38	36	36	35	33	33	32	31
19 / 4 / 122	53	51	49	48	46	45	43	42	41	40	39	38	36	36	35	33	33	32	31
19 / 6 / 123	53	51	50	48	46	45	44	43	41	40	39	38	37	36	35	34	33	32	31
19 / 8 / 124	54	52	50	48	47	46	44	43	41	40	39	38	37	36	35	34	33	32	32
19 / 10 / 125	54	52	51	49	47	46	44	43	42	41	39	39	37	37	35	34	34	33	32
19 / 12 / 126	55	52	51	49	47	46	45	44	42	41	40	39	38	37	36	35	34	33	32
20 / 0 / 127	55	53	52	50	48	47	45	44	42	41	40	39	38	37	36	35	34	33	32
20 / 2 / 128	55	53	52	50	48	47	45	44	43	42	40	40	38	37	36	35	34	33	33
20 / 4 / 129	56	54	52	50	49	47	46	45	43	42	41	40	39	38	36	35	34	33	33
20 / 6 / 130	56	54	53	51	49	48	46	45	43	42	41	40	39	38	37	36	35	34	33
20 / 8 / 131	57	55	53	51	49	48	46	45	43	42	41	40	39	38	37	36	35	34	33
20 / 10 / 132	57	55	54	52	50	48	47	46	44	43	42	41	39	39	37	36	35	34	34
20 / 12 / 132	57	55	54	52	50	48	47	46	44	43	42	41	39	39	37	36	35	34	34

BMI <18.4 = underweight; BMI 18.5–24.9 = acceptable; BMI 25–29.9 = overweight; BMI 30–39.9 = obese; BMI >40 = morbidly obese

Appendix 5

ESTIMATION OF RENAL FUNCTION

Various formulae have been devised to estimate renal function, but the two that are most commonly used are:

- Cockcroft and Gault equation;
- Modified Diet in Renal Disease (MDRD) equation – commonly known as eGFR (estimated glomerular filtration rate).

Both of these equations rely on measurement of **serum creatinine**. Creatinine is a muscle breakdown product and the serum concentration of creatinine will not change from day to day because the rate of production is constant and is equal to the rate at which it is eliminated from the body by the kidneys. Thus **creatinine clearance** is used as a measure of the **glomerular filtration rate (GFR)** and hence renal function. Various factors affect serum creatinine, including muscle mass, sex, age, weight and race, and these need to be taken into account.

One major difference between the two equations is that the MDRD equation predicts GFR for a standard body surface area (BSA) of $1.73\,m^2$ (i.e. the patient's weight is not needed). This is the reason why most hospital pathology laboratories use the MDRD equation as they only need to know the serum creatinine value.

The Cockcroft and Gault equation predicts a non-normalized creatinine clearance as it takes into account the patient's weight, i.e. it measures what the kidneys are actually doing.

eGFR values are increasingly being reported by hospital laboratories in place of serum creatinine.

When looking at estimations of renal function, it is important to know which calculation has been used to determine GFR – eGFR can give a lower value. In addition, the dosing recommendations for drugs used in renal impairment found in reference books and manufacturers' data sheets are based on the Cockcroft and Gault equation. Taking these two facts into account, it is recommended that the **Cockcroft and Gault equation should be used when adjusting drug doses to an individual's renal function.**

Therefore, we will look at the use of the Cockcroft and Gault equation in more detail.

Cockcroft and Gault suggested the following formula, which applies to **adults aged 20+:**

For **men:**

$$\text{CrCl (mL/min)} = \frac{1.23 \times (140 - \text{age}) \times \text{weight}}{\text{serum creatinine (mcmol/L)}}$$

$$= \frac{(140 - \text{age}) \times \text{weight}}{\text{serum creatinine (mg/100 mL)}}$$

For **women:**

TIP BOX

Ensure that the correct value and units for serum creatinine are used.

WORKED EXAMPLE

Calculate the creatinine clearance of a male patient aged 67 years, weight 72 kg, having a serum creatinine of 125 mcmol/L.

As the units of the serum creatinine are given in mcmol, we must ensure that the right formula is used, i.e.:

$$\text{CrCl (mL/min)} = \frac{1.23 \times (140 - \text{age}) \times \text{weight}}{\text{serum creatinine (mcmol/L)}}$$

where:

$$\text{age (years)} = 67$$
$$\text{weight (kg)} = 72$$
$$\text{serum creatinine (mcmol/L)} = 125$$

Substituting the figures into the formula:

TIP BOX

In the top line, the sum within the brackets is done first, i.e. $(140 - 67)$, then multiply by 1.23 and then by 72: $(140 - 67) = 73$, so the sum becomes $1.23 \times 73 \times 72 = 6,464.88$.

Appendix 6

ABBREVIATIONS USED IN PRESCRIPTIONS

Although directions should preferably be in English without abbreviations, it is recognized that some Latin abbreviations are still used.

The following is a list of common English abbreviations and Latin abbreviations that are commonly used. It should be noted that the English versions are not exact translations.

NOTE Some of these abbreviations may differ as they depend upon local convention.

ABBREVIATION	LATIN DERIVATION	ENGLISH MEANING
a.c.	*ante cibum*	before food
alt die	*alterna die*	alternate days
appli	*applicatio*	an application
aurist.	*auristillae*	ear drops
b.d. (BD)	*bis die*	twice daily
b.i.d. (BID)	*bis in die*	twice a day
c or c̄	*cum*	with
c.c.	*cum cibum*	with food (also: cubic centimetre)
crem	*cremor*	a cream
D	*dies*	daily
Elix		elixir
gtt (g)	*guttae*	drops
H	*hors*	hour/at the hour of
h.s.	*hora somni*	at bedtime (lit: at the hour of sleep)
INH		inhaler/to be inhaled
Inj		an injection
IM		intramuscular
Irrig	*irrigatio*	an irrigation
IV		intravenously
IU		International Units
M	*mane*	(in the) morning
m.d.u.	*more dictus utendus*	to be used or taken as directed

mist	*mistura*	mixture
mitte		please dispense (lit: send)
N	*nocte*	(at) night
NEB		nebules/to be nebulized
O	*omni*	every
oculent (oc)	*oculentum*	eye ointment
o.d. (OD)	*omni die*	every day (daily)
o.m. (OM)	*omni mane*	every morning
o.n. (ON)	*omni nocte*	every night
p.c. (PC)	*post cibum*	after food
p.o. (PO)	*per os*	orally (by mouth)
p.r. (PR)	*per rectum*	rectally
p.r.n. (PRN)	*pro re nata*	occasionally (when required0
p.v. (PV)	*per vagina*	vaginally
Q	*quaque*	each/every
		(e.g. q6h = every 6 hours)
q.i.d. (QID)	*quarter in die*	four times a day
q.d.s. (QDS)	*quater die sumendus*	to be taken four times a day
Rx		'recipe' = take
S		without
Sig	*signa*	let it be labelled
SC		subcutaneous
SL		sublingual
s.o.s.	*si opus sit*	if required
Stat	*statum*	at once
supp *or* suppos	*suppositorium*	a suppository
TDD		total daily dose
t.i.d. (TID)	*ter in die*	three times a day
t.d.s. (TDS)	*ter die sumendus*	to be taken three times a day
TOP		topically
U *or* UN		units
Ung	*unguentum*	an ointment

INDEX

Note: page numbers in **bold** refer to figures, page numbers in *italics* refer to information contained in tables.